ASPECTS IN CONTINUOUS RENAL REPLACEMENT THERAPY

Edited by **Ayman Karkar**

Aspects in Continuous Renal Replacement Therapy

http://dx.doi.org/10.5772/intechopen.76484
Edited by Ayman Karkar

Contributors

Sandip Mitra, Patrick Hamilton, Rhodri Harris, Somchai Eiam-Ong, Kullaya Takkavatakarn, Paweena Susantitaphong, Jorge Echeverri, Carolina Larrarte, Manuel Huerfano, Ahmed Alkhunaizi, Ayman Karkar

First published in London, United Kingdom, 2019 by IntechOpen
IntechOpen is the global imprint of INTECHOPEN LIMITED, registered in England and Wales, registration number: 11086078, The Shard, 25th floor, 32 London Bridge Street
London, SE19SG – United Kingdom
Printed in Croatia

British Library Cataloguing-in-Publication Data
A catalogue record for this book is available from the British Library

Additional hard copies can be obtained from orders@intechopen.com

Aspects in Continuous Renal Replacement Therapy, Edited by Ayman Karkar
p. cm.
Print ISBN 978-1-78985-585-2
Online ISBN 978-1-78985-586-9

For EU product safety concerns:
IN TECH d.o.o., Prolaz Marije Krucifikse Kozulić 3, 51000 Rijeka, Croatia,
info@intechopen.com or visit our website at intechopen.com.

Meet the editor

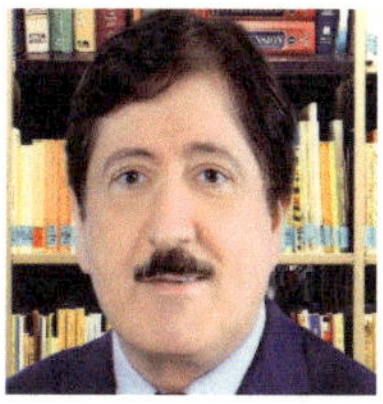

Following his graduation from medical school, Dr. Ayman Karkar received his MSc degree in Nephrology and Hypertension and his PhD degree in Renal Medicine from Hammersmith Hospital, University of London. Dr. Karkar is a consultant physician and nephrologist, Fellow of the Royal Colleges of Physicians of London, Edinburgh, Glasgow, and Ireland, and Fellow of the American National Kidney Foundation and the American Society of Nephrology. He has authored several books and book chapters and published over 150 articles and abstracts in peer-reviewed medical journals. Dr. Karkar is currently Baxter Head of Medical Affairs—Renal Care, Middle East and Africa, and Subject Matter Expert, East and Central Europe and Middle East and Africa.

Contents

Preface

Continuous renal replacement therapy (CRRT) has witnessed significant improvement since the technique was implemented by Peter Kramer of Göttingen (Germany) in 1977. The technique was established when Kramer was trying to introduce a catheter into the femoral vein for initiating hemodialysis. Accidently, the catheter went into the femoral artery, but Kramer realized the value of the arterial-venous pressure difference (i.e. blood flow driven by mean arterial pressure) in providing an ultrafiltration and convection/hemofiltration concept and the need of replacement solutions, which came to be known as "continuous arterio-venous hemofiltration." Later, in 1987, Peter Robert Uldall (Toronto, Canada) introduced "continuous veno-venous hemofiltration" by providing a pump and replacing the need for arterial pressure; a technique that avoided the potential risks and complications of puncturing a major artery and the possible slow or altered blood flow rates due to frequent hypotension in critically ill or shocked patients.

CRRT is a slow and smooth continuous extracorporeal blood purification process. It is usually implemented over 24 hours to several days with gentle removal of fluid overload and excess uremic toxins. CRRT has benefited lately from significant improvements in technology and quality performance in managing critically ill patients with acute kidney injury, brain injury, and/or multiorgan failure in intensive care units. These advancements include improved monitor technology, medical devices (dialyzers and adsorbers), disposables, and a variety of different compositions of replacement solutions. *Aspects in CRRT* covers selected and important topics in CRRT. These are "Principles and methods of acute therapies," "Acute kidney injury," "Hemodiafiltration in acute kidney injury," "Immunoadsorption techniques and their current role in the intensive care unit," and "CRRT specialized teams." Each of these chapters provides a clear description in a simple and easily understood layout. All chapters are well referenced and updated, and supported by clear figures and tables. *Aspects in CRRT* is written by distinguished and experienced authors, and their tremendous efforts and valued contributions are much appreciated.

Finally, my special thanks go to the Author Service Managers Ms. Danijela Sakic and Ms. Marija Gojevic-Zrnic for their great efforts and professional secretarial expertise in collecting and editing the manuscripts.

Ayman Karkar
Consultant Physician and Nephrologist
Baxter Head of Medical Affairs—Renal Care, Middle East and Africa
Baxter International, Deerfield, USA

Chapter 1

Introductory Chapter: Principles and Methods of Acute Therapies

Ayman Karkar

Additional information is available at the end of the chapter

http://dx.doi.org/10.5772/intechopen.82503

1. Introduction

Continuous renal replacement therapy (CRRT) is a slow and smooth continuous extracorporeal blood purification. CRRT is usually implemented over 24 h to several days with an aim of gentle removal of fluid overload and excess uremic toxins, where the continuous filtration simulates the continuity of kidney functions. It is usually indicated in critically ill and hemodynamically unstable (adult and pediatric) patients with acute kidney injury (AKI) and/or multiorgan failure, sepsis/shock, acute brain injury, or other causes of increased intracranial pressure or generalized brain edema in intensive care unit (ICU), where such patients cannot tolerate the relatively fast removal of fluids (and solutes) by conventional hemodialysis (HD).

Continuous renal replacement therapy witnessed significant improvement since the technique was implemented by Peter Kramer of Göttingen (Germany) in 1977 [1]. The technique was established when Kramer was trying to introduce a catheter into the femoral vein for initiating HD. Accidently, the catheter went into the femoral artery, when Kramer realized the value of the arterial-venous pressure difference (i.e., blood flow driven by mean arterial pressure) in providing ultrafiltration and convection/hemofiltration concept and the need of replacement solutions, which was known as "continuous arterio-venous hemofiltration (CAVH)". Later, in 1987, Peter Robert Uldall (Toronto, Canada) [2] introduced the "continuous veno-venous hemofiltration (CVVH)" by providing a pump and replacing the need of the arterial pressure, a technique that avoided (a) the potential risks and complications of puncturing a major artery (e.g., infection, distal thrombosis, and disconnection/bleeding) and (b) the possible slow or altered blood flow rates due to frequent hypotension in critically ill or shocked patients.

Continuous renal replacement therapy is based on four main physiologic principles. These are (a) diffusion, (b) ultrafiltration, (c) convection, and (d) adsorption. In clinical practice, there is more than one principle implemented in achieving the goals of required treatment (e.g., diffusion, ultrafiltration, and convection). CRRT can be performed in one or more of the following four modalities: (1) slow continuous ultrafiltration (SCUF), (2) continuous veno-venous hemofiltration (CVVH), (3) continuous veno-venous hemodiafiltration (CVVHDF), and (4) continuous veno-venous hemodialysis (CVVHD). Other therapeutic modalities that can be used in conjunction with CRRT include therapeutic plasma exchange and hemoperfusion/adsorption.

The performance and delivery of CRRT depends on an efficient vascular access (e.g., internal jugular or femoral vein), specifically designed HD machines and high-flux membranes/dialyzers. Synthetic and biocompatible membranes/dialyzers are capable of efficiently removing excess fluids and clearing small and middle-larger-size uremic toxins [3], and some have high adsorptive affinity to proteins, endotoxins, and inflammatory mediators (e.g., cytokines) [4]. Following high convective volume of ultrafiltration, the replacement/substitution solutions, which can be infused before (predilution) or after the dialyzer (postdilution), are sterile physiological fluids [5] that consist of balanced electrolyte solutions of either lactate or bicarbonate base, which resembles the composition of the ultrafiltrate (but without the removed uremic wastes). The long duration of this extracorporeal blood purification technique, where the blood is in direct contact with blood tubes and dialyzer membrane for longer period than conventional HD, requires continuous anticoagulation to prevent clotting and extend the circuit life. Heparin has been widely used, but it has been associated with increased risk of bleeding. Regional citrate anticoagulation (RCA) is the more preferred and recommended method of anticoagulation, where it has been associated with significantly less bleeding [6], less blood transfusion [7], and extended life of the extracorporeal circuit [8].

Initiation of CRRT is indicated in patients with (a) hemodynamic instability/shock, (b) diuretic-resistant fluid overload, (c) severe metabolic acidosis ($pH < 7.2$), and (d) refractory hyperkalemia ($K+ > 6.5$). CRRT has also been considered in drug toxicity and in prevention of radiocontrast-induced nephropathy [5]. The goals of CRRT include (i) clearance of uremic toxins, (ii) correction of electrolytes disturbance, (iii) acid-base balance, (iv) hemodynamic stabilization, (v) fluid balance, (vi) nutritional support, and (vii) removal and/or modulation of inflammatory mediators in septic patients. The success of CRRT depends on the prescribed and achieved dose of replacement/substitution fluids, treatment duration, type of dialyzer, and method and dose of anticoagulation, in addition to a well-established CRRT management protocol (e.g., type, size, length, placement and care of central lines, indications, when to start, and when to stop CRRT). Furthermore, the delivery and performance of CRRT requires well-trained medical and nursing staff.

Despite the general safety and valuable advantages, CRRT has some limitations. These include the requirement of a large-bore central vascular access (a risk source of infection), hypotension (decreased organ perfusion), continuous anticoagulation (inappropriate doses or inadequate control of anticoagulants may lead to bleeding, which is associated with a decrease in hemoglobin level and/or drop in blood pressure and possible need of blood transfusion, or clot formation that is associated with short circuit life, interruption of prescribed dose, inadequate therapy, and increased cost), electrolyte imbalance (potassium, phosphorus, and magnesium), drug removal (e.g., antibiotics), and immobilization of the patient for prolonged periods [9].

However, most of these limitations can either be prevented or be controlled [10]. A drop-in blood pressure, though much less encountered than in intermittent HD, is usually compensated for by the patient or, in some cases, requires inotropic support to maintain effective mean arterial pressure. Furthermore, CRRT prescription can be modified at any time during treatment based on hemodynamic situation. A well-established protocol of RCA, for example, can help in maintaining the patency of the extracorporeal circuit for a longer period and in avoiding uncontrolled bleeding. Implementation of infection control policies and procedures, including aseptic techniques, can help in preventing or reducing the vascular access catheter-associated infection. Regular monitoring and assessment of electrolytes and blood gases and the selection of appropriate replacement solutions (e.g., bicarbonate-based buffer and required composition of electrolytes and supplements) not only can help in replacing plasma volume removed by ultrafiltration but can also ensure the correction of electrolyte and acid-base imbalances. Drug removal in CRRT depends on its molecular weight, the sieving coefficient, and the degree of protein binding. Drugs with significant protein binding are removed minimally. Some drugs may be removed by adsorption to the membrane. Most of the commonly used drugs, including antibiotics, require monitoring and dose adjustments [11]. Finally, CRRT patients are prone to hypothermia due to the significant volume of blood that is circulated outside the body, and the significant volumes of the substitution and dialysate fluid used. Although newer CRRT machines are equipped with blood warmers that can bring both dialysate and substitution fluids to 37°C (98.6°F), a close monitoring of body temperature of patients is recommended especially when larger volumes of substitution and dialysate solutions are used.

2. Conclusions

Severe acute kidney injury, especially when it is caused or associated with sepsis, carries increased risk of progression to chronic kidney disease and end-stage renal failure. In addition, it is associated with prolonged hospitalization, financial burden, and increased mortality rate. Critically ill patients with acute kidney injury and/or multiorgan failure in ICU require special modalities of therapies to ensure hemodynamic stability, euvolemic status, and acid-base and electrolytes balance with an aim of speeding up renal recovery and avoiding deleterious consequences. CRRT stands as a valuable supportive therapeutic modality for such patients. CRRT management includes specific indications, adequate prescription, timing of initiation and termination, proper anticoagulation, and removal of endotoxins and inflammatory mediators in different settings of associated sepsis.

Disclosures

No funding sources and relevant disclosures to declare.

Author details

Ayman Karkar

Address all correspondence to: han94dan97@gmail.com

Baxter AG, Dubai, United Arab Emirates

References

[1] Kramer P, Wigger W, Reiger J, Matthaei D, Scheler F. Arteriovenous haemofiltration: A new and simple method for treatment of overhydrated patients resistant to diuretics [in German]. Klinische Wochenschrift. 1977;**55**:1121-1122

[2] deVeber GA. Peter Robert Uldall 1935-1995. Nephrology, Dialysis, Transplantation. 1996; **11**:902-903 https://renal.org/about-the-renal-association/history/obituaries/peter-robert-uldall/

[3] Karkar A. Introductory Chapter to "Aspects in Dialysis" Book. Editor: Ayman Karkar. Rijeka: Intech. ISBN 978-1-78923-025-3. https://www.intechopen.com/books/aspects-in-dialysis

[4] Malard B, Lambert C, Kellum JA. In vitro comparison of the adsorption of inflammatory mediators by blood purification devices. Intensive Care Medicine Experimental. 2018;**6**:12. DOI: 10.1186/s40635-018-0177-2

[5] KDIGO Acute Kidney Injury Work Group. Kidney International. Supplement. 2012; **2**:1-138

[6] Bai M, Zhou M, He L, Ma F, Li YY, Wang P, et al. Citrate versus heparin anticoagulation for continuous renal replacement therapy: An updated meta-analysis of RCTs. ICM. 2015;**41**(12):2098-2110

[7] Borg R, Ugboma D, Walker DM, Partridge R. Evaluating the safety and efficacy of regional citrate compared to systemic heparin as anticoagulation for continuous renal replacement therapy in critically ill patients: A service evaluation following a change in practice. Journal of the Intensive Care Soceity. 2017;**18**(3):184-192

[8] Zhang Z, Hongying N. Efficacy and safety of regional citrate anticoagulation in critically ill patients undergoing continuous renal replacement therapy. ICM. 2012;**38**(1):20-28

[9] Clark WR, Neri M, Garzotto F, Ricci Z, Goldstein SL, Ding X, et al. The future of critical care: Renal support in 2027. Critical Care. 2017;**21**:92. DOI: 10.1186/s13054-017-1665-6

[10] Sigwalt F, Bouteleux A, Dambricourt F, Asselborn T, Moriceau F, Rimmelé T. Clinical complications of continuous renal replacement therapy. Contributions to Nephrology. 2018;**194**:109-117

[11] Lewis SJ, Mueller BA. Antibiotics dosing in critically ill patients receiving CRRT: Under dosing is over prevalent. Seminars in Dialysis. 2014;**27**(5):441-445

Chapter 2

Acute Kidney Injury

Ahmed M. Alkhunaizi

Additional information is available at the end of the chapter

http://dx.doi.org/10.5772/intechopen.80625

Abstract

Acute kidney injury (AKI), previously named acute renal failure, is characterized by abrupt deterioration in renal function. The incidence of AKI has increased lately, both in the hospital and community setting. It is estimated that more than 13 million people are affected by AKI annually worldwide. Despite all the advances in the field, AKI still carries a high mortality rate. In addition to mortality, AKI is an important risk factor for the development of chronic kidney disease. In this chapter, various aspects of AKI will be discussed including definition and staging, etiology, pathophysiology, clinical presentation, diagnosis, management, prognosis, and prevention.

Keywords: acute kidney injury, renal failure, nephrotoxicity, pathophysiology, biomarkers, management, prognosis, prevention

1. Introduction

Acute kidney injury (AKI) is a major public health concern and is associated with high morbidity, mortality, and healthcare costs. The incidence of AKI has increased lately, both in the hospital and community setting. It is estimated that more than 13 million people are affected by AKI annually with an incidence of 21.6% in adults and 33.7% in children during a single hospital episode of care [1, 2]. Despite all the advances in the field, the mortality of AKI remains very high estimated at 23.9% in adults and 13.8% in children [2]. In addition to the high mortality (1.7 million per year), AKI is associated with high morbidity and high costs [1]. In the United States, at least $5 billion in hospital costs are related to AKI, while in England AKI consumes 1% of the National Health Service budget [3]. In the developed world, AKI manifests mainly in older patients and in the intensive care settings; while in the developing countries, adults and women are particularly more commonly affected [4, 5]. Recovery from AKI is not always, as previously thought, complete and many patients progress to develop chronic kidney disease (CKD), end-stage renal disease (ESRD), or worsening of preexisting CKD later on in life [6–9]. Treatment of AKI is needed to reduce the high morbidity and mortality and improve recovery of renal function. A part of dialysis, there are no other interventions that reliably improve survival, limit injury, or enhance recovery. The multifactorial etiology and the heterogeneous patient population coupled with the complicated clinical course of patients with AKI has created challenges in the search for effective pharmacological therapy [10]. In some scenarios, such as surgery or administration of intravenous contrast, the onset of AKI can be predicted providing a window of opportunity for intervention and prevention. In the majority of cases, however, intervention takes place after the onset of AKI with the aim to shorten the course and enhance recovery of renal function. In this chapter, various aspects of AKI will be discussed with a particular focus on definition and staging, etiology, pathophysiology, clinical presentation, diagnosis, management, prognosis, and prevention.

2. Definition and staging of acute kidney injury

The term AKI has replaced old terms such as acute renal failure and acute renal insufficiency, which previously had been used to describe the same clinical condition. AKI is not just failure; it also incorporates the entire spectrum of the syndrome, from minor changes in renal function to the most severe form, where renal replacement therapy (RRT) may be required.

Over the last few decades, more than 35 different definitions have been used to define AKI [11]. The most commonly used definition is based on urine output and/or serum creatinine criteria. The most commonly used classifications of AKI are the "risk, injury, failure, loss of kidney function, and end-stage kidney disease" (RIFLE) [12] and the Acute Kidney Injury Network (AKIN) classifications [13].

The RIFLE classification is based on serum creatinine and urine output determinants, and considers three severity classes of AKI (risk, injury and failure), according to the variations in serum creatinine and or urine output, and two outcome classes (loss of kidney function and end-stage kidney disease). The patient should be classified using the criteria which leads to the

Class	GFR	Urine output
Risk	↑ SCr × 1.5 or ↓ GFR >25%	<0.5 mL/kg/h × 6 h
Injury	↑ SCr × 2 or ↓ GFR >50%	<0.5 mL/kg/h × 12 h
Failure	↑ SCr × 3 or ↓ GFR >75% or if baseline SCr ≥353.6 μmol/L (≥4 mg/dL) ↑ SCr >44.2 μmol/L (>0.5 mg/dL)	<0.3 mL/kg/h × 24 h or anuria × 12 h
Loss of kidney function	Complete loss of kidney function >4 weeks	
End-stage kidney disease	Complete loss of kidney function >3 months	

GFR, glomerular filtration rate; SCr, serum creatinine.

Table 1. Risk, injury, failure, loss of kidney function and end-stage kidney disease (RIFLE) classification of acute kidney injury [12].

http://dx.doi.org/10.5772/intechopen.80625

worst classification (maximum RIFLE), **Table 1**. On the other hand, AKI is classified/staged by the AKIN into three stages as shown in **Table 2**.

The Kidney Disease Improving Global Outcomes (KDIGO) work group has combined the RIFLE and AKIN classifications in order to establish one classification of AKI for practice, research and public health. Therefore, AKI is now defined as an abrupt reduction in renal function (within 48 h) based on an increase in serum creatinine level of more than or equal to 0.3 mg/dL (≥26.4 μmol/L), a percentage increase in serum creatinine of more than or equal to 50% (1.5-fold from baseline), or a reduction in urine output (documented oliguria of less than 0.5 mL/kg/h for more than 6 h) or a combination of these factors [14].

Stage	Change in serum creatinine	Urine output
1	Increase ≥0.3 mg/dL (26.52 μmol/L) or ≥150–200% from baseline	<0.5 mL/kg/h for more than 6 h
2	Increase >200–300% from baseline	<0.5 mL/kg/h for more than 12 h
3	Increase >300% from baseline or ≥4.0 mg/dL (353.60 μmol/L) with an acute rise of at least 0.5 mg/dL (44.20 μmol/L)	<0.3 mL/kg/h for 24 h or anuria for 12 h

Table 2. Acute Kidney Injury Network (AKIN) classifications of acute kidney injury [13].

3. Etiology of acute kidney injury

The etiology of AKI can be divided into three categories, **Table 3** [15]:

1. Prerenal (caused by decreased renal perfusion, often due to volume depletion)
2. Intrinsic renal (caused by a process within the kidneys)
3. Postrenal (caused by a process distal to the kidneys such as obstruction)

Prerenal

Intrarenal vasoconstriction (hemodynamically mediated):

Medications: nonsteroidal anti-inflammatory drugs, angiotensin system blockers, calcineurin inhibitors

Cardiorenal syndrome: advanced heart failure

Hepatorenal syndrome: liver cirrhosis

Abdominal compartment syndrome

Hypercalcemia

Systemic vasodilation: sepsis

Volume depletion:

Renal loss: diuretics, osmotic diuresis (severe hyperglycemia), salt wasting

Extrarenal loss: blood loss, gastrointestinal loss (vomiting, diarrhea), skin (burns, sweating)

Intrinsic renal

Glomerulonephritis (isolated or a part of systemic diseases)

Interstitial nephritis:

Medications: antibiotics (β lactams, sulfonamides, quinolones, rifampin), phenytoin, antiretrovirals, proton pump inhibitors, nonsteroidal anti-inflammatory drugs

Infections: viruses (Epstein-Barr virus, cytomegalovirus, human immunodeficiency virus), bacteria (tuberculosis, legionella species), fungi (candidiasis, histoplasmosis)

Systemic disease: sarcoidosis, connective tissue diseases

Tubular necrosis:

Ischemic: prolonged hypotension

Nephrotoxic: exogenous toxins (radiographic contrast agents, aminoglycosides, cisplatin, methotrexate, amphotericin B)

Endogenous toxins: pigment induced (hemolysis and rhabdomyolysis), tumor lysis syndrome, multiple myeloma

Vascular

Renal artery and vein thrombosis, malignant hypertension, scleroderma renal crisis, atheroembolic disease, microangiopathies

Post renal

Extrarenal obstruction: outlet obstruction (prostate hypertrophy, neurogenic bladder; malignancy of the urogenital tract), retroperitoneal fibrosis

Intrarenal obstruction: stones, crystals (acyclovir, indinavir, ethylene glycol), blood clots, tumors

Adapted and modified from Rahman et al. [15].

Table 3. Etiology of acute kidney injury.

Of these three categories, only "intrinsic" AKI represents a true kidney disease, while pre- and postrenal AKI are the consequence of extrarenal processes that lead to decreased glomerular filtration rate (GFR). Both pre- and postrenal conditions, if persist and not managed in a timely manner, may eventually evolve into intrinsic renal damage. Patients with CKD and those admitted to the intensive care unit (ICU) are particularly prone to develop AKI. The AKI-EPI study demonstrated that AKI occurred in more than half of the patients in ICU; mostly due to sepsis and hypovolemia followed by nephrotoxic agents [16].

4. Pathophysiology of acute kidney injury

Despite the identification of several cellular mechanisms thought to underlie the development of AKI, the pathophysiology of AKI is still poorly understood. Animal models of AKI representing ischemia–reperfusion injury and drug nephrotoxicity have been instrumental in understanding the pathophysiology of AKI in humans. Although the current *in vivo* models of AKI in healthy rodents provide valuable information about the pathophysiological mechanisms of renal injury, they do not reflect the complexity of disease in humans characterized by population's heterogeneity and preexisting comorbidities such as diabetes, hypertension, and CKD. A few and not all mechanisms of AKI will be discussed.

4.1. Microvascular injury

The renal microvasculature plays a key role in the pathophysiology of AKI. The kidney is a vascular organ receiving 25% of the cardiac output and has a high energy demand with relatively low oxygen (O_2) extraction. Under normal steady-state, the O_2 supply to the kidney is well regulated. Adequate O_2 delivery is crucial for the production of mitochondrial adenosine triphosphate (ATP), nitric oxide (NO), and reactive oxygen species (ROS) necessary for homeostatic control of renal function [10, 17]. The vascular architecture of the outer medulla is particularly susceptible to ischemic injury due to the marginal oxygenation of this part of the kidney.

With injury, the microcirculation is compromised leading to an imbalance in NO, ROS, and O_2 supply and consumption. Subsequent pathogenic events follow including hypoxia and oxidative stress. Injury to the microvascular endothelium and changes in the glycocalyx lead to endothelial cell activation and expression of cell surface markers that promote recruitment and adhesion of leukocytes and platelets, leading to further changes in perfusion and O_2 delivery; and to additional endothelial cell injury and inflammation [18, 19]. As a result, increased vascular permeability and development of interstitial edema lead to further compromise of blood flow exacerbating the initial insult. In addition, production of vasoactive prostaglandins by damaged tubular cells coupled with oxidative stress further impairs O_2 delivery by worsening the local microvascular occlusion [18, 19]. The main long-term result of microvascular injury is a reduction in peritubular capillary density, a response to decreased vascular endothelial growth factor (VEGF) and increased transforming growth factor beta (TGF-β) signaling, which contributes to ongoing hypoxia and development of renal fibrosis [20].

4.2. Changes in endoplasmic reticulum

The endoplasmic reticulum (ER) plays an important role in the maintenance of protein homeostasis through its control of the concentration, conformation, folding, and trafficking of client proteins. As a result of endothelial or epithelial cell stress, unfolded or misfolded proteins accumulate in the ER, triggering the unfolded protein response (UPR) [21]. The UPR initially serves as an adaptive response, but will also induce apoptosis in cells under severe or prolonged ER stress. Accumulating evidence indicates that apoptosis in tubules resulting from epithelial cell damage is caused, at least in part, by the proapoptotic UPR [22]. Therefore, targeting the UPR may present a possible approach to prevent or treat AKI.

4.3. Mitochondrial dysfunction

The ER and mitochondria have multiple contact sites termed the mitochondrial-ER-associated membrane (MAM). The MAM contains proteins from the two organelles and appears as ER tubules closely apposed to the mitochondria on electron micrographs [23]. During cellular stress situations, like an altered cellular redox state, the MAM alters its set of regulatory proteins and thus alters MAM functions. In the pathogenesis of AKI, proximal tubules are especially vulnerable to mitochondrial dysfunction as they depend on aerobic metabolism and their mitochondria are in a more oxidized state than those in the distal tubular cells which can use glycolysis [24]. Following either ATP depletion or cisplatin treatment of rat renal tubular cells, mitochondrial fragmentation was observed prior to cytochrome c release and apoptosis [25]. Targeting mitochondrial dysfunction along with a better understanding of the regulation of mitochondrial dynamics and its pathogenic changes may emerge as a new modality to treat AKI [26].

4.4. Autophagy

Autophagy is a catabolic process in which proteins, organelles, and cytoplasmic components are delivered to lysosomes for degradation and recycling. Autophagy is induced in renal tubular cells during AKI [27]. It is initiated by encapsulating cytoplasmic proteins and organelles in autophagosomes, which fuse with lysosomes for degradation. Once activated, it may decrease cellular stress by removing ER membranes containing UPR sensors and/or clearing abnormal proteins from the ER. In animal models, blocking the autophagic flux-enhanced AKI, while activation of autophagy was found to be protective against cisplatin-induced AKI [27]. In addition, resolution of autophagy may promote proliferation and regeneration of tubular cells in the recovery phase of AKI [28]. Autophagy may be targeted as an inflammatory modulator for the treatment of various kidney diseases [29].

4.5. Inflammation

Inflammation plays a major role in the pathophysiology of AKI resulting from ischemia [30]. Changes in protein folding and mitochondrial function influence the innate immune response, contributing to inflammation. In addition, several cytokines and inflammatory pathways are activated in AKI [30]. Moreover, immune cells of both the innate and adaptive immune systems, such as neutrophils, dendritic cells, macrophages, and lymphocytes, contribute to the pathogenesis of renal injury after ischemia–reperfusion injury, and some cells also participate in the repair process [31]. Neutrophils and monocytes mediate the acute phase within the first 24 h of injury [32], whereas T and B lymphocytes are important in the evolution phase of renal injury [31]. Inhibition of leukocyte infiltration into the kidney ameliorates the loss in renal function, decreases renal injury, cell death, and long-term fibrosis [33]. There is experimental evidence that inducible nitric oxide synthase (iNOS) may contribute to tubular injury during AKI [34]. It has been shown that hypoxia in isolated proximal tubules increases nitric oxide release [35], and that iNOS protein expression is increased in ischemic kidneys [36]. *In vivo* use of an antisense oligonucleotide to block the up-regulation of iNOS was protective against ischemia induced renal injury in rat models [36]. Similarly, tubules from iNOS knockout mice were protected against hypoxic injury [37].

Phospholipase A2 (PLA2) is a family of enzymes that hydrolyzes the acyl group from the sn-2 position of phospholipids, generating free fatty acids [38, 39]. PLA2 activity is increased during hypoxic injury to the renal tubules. Inhibiting PLA2 by exogenous fatty acids such as arachidonic acid has been shown to be protective against hypoxia-induced injury in isolated proximal renal tubules [40, 41].

4.6. Sepsis and acute kidney injury

Sepsis is a severe inflammatory response to infection characterized by a whole-body inflammatory state with severe consequences, including multiple organ failure [42]. AKI is a frequent and serious complication of sepsis among ICU patients and is associated with a high in-hospital and long-term mortality [43, 44]. The multinational AKI-EPI study has demonstrated that AKI affected more than 50% of ICU patients, and increasing AKI severity was associated with increased mortality [16].

4.6.1. Pathogenesis of sepsis-induced acute kidney injury

Although septic shock is a leading cause of AKI, the underlying mechanisms are not completely understood. The pathophysiology of AKI in sepsis is complex and multifactorial involving multiple processes including intrarenal hemodynamic perturbations, endothelial dysfunction, infiltration of inflammatory cells, up-regulation of inflammatory cytokines, intraglomerular thrombosis, induction of apoptosis, and tubular obstruction with necrotic cells and debris [42, 45, 46]. Activation of pro- and anti-inflammatory mechanisms is believed to play a key role in the induction of sepsis [47].

Activation of the innate immune response takes place after initial host-microbial encounter, which coordinates a defensive response involving both humoral and cellular components [48]. This leads to activation and secretion of various cytokines, most importantly interleukin-1 (IL-1), tumor necrosis factor-α (TNF-α), and IL-6 that progress to a state of cytokine storm, hemodynamic instability, and eventually organ dysfunction and septic shock [42].

Lipopolysaccharide (LPS), a component of the outer membrane of Gram-negative bacteria, is a potent and rapid activator of a variety of cell types such as leukocytes, monocytes, and macrophages [49]. Activation of inflammatory cells by LPS constitutes the first step in a cascade of events that lead to the manifestation of Gram-negative sepsis. LPS initiates multiple intracellular signaling events, including the activation of nuclear factor-κB (NF-κB), which ultimately leads to the synthesis and release of a number of pro-inflammatory mediators, including IL-1, IL-6,IL-8, and TNF-a. The pathway that leads to activation of NF-κB has been shown to be mediated by members of the toll-like receptors (TLRs), a family of transmembrane proteins that play an important role in the defense against pathogenic microbial infection [50]. In the setting of sepsis, there is a significant up-regulation of TLRs, in particular TLR-2 and TLR-4 expression [51]. Both TLR-2 and TLR-4 are activated by LPS in a response that depends on LPS-binding protein and is enhanced by CD14 [49, 52]. An overview of the TLR signaling pathway is depicted in **Figure 1** [53]. **Figure 2** depicts the key pathways involved in the clinical course of sepsis that also have implications in the pathophysiology of sepsis-induced AKI [42].

Modulation of TLRs may become a novel therapeutic target in the treatment of organ dysfunction associated with sepsis including AKI. Similarly, cytokine adsorption to the membrane during continuous renal replacement therapy may emerge as a treatment modality in patients with sepsis and AKI [54].

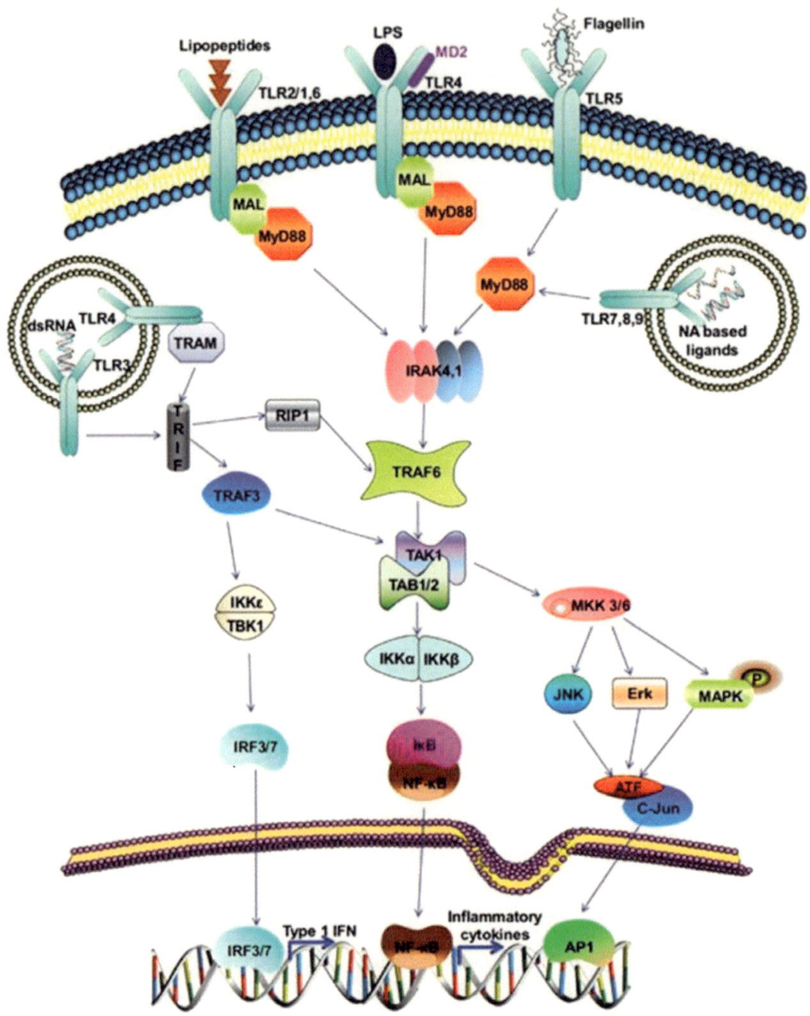

Figure 1. Toll-like receptor (TLR) signaling pathway. When TLRs are stimulated by their respective ligands, they dimerize and recruit downstream adaptor molecules, such as myeloid differentiation primary-response protein 88 (MyD88), MyD88-adaptor-like (MAL), toll/interleukin (IL)-1 receptor (TIR)-domain-containing adaptor-inducing interferon-β (TRIF), TRIF-related adaptor molecule (TRAM), which activate other downstream molecules leading to the activation of signaling cascades that converge at the nuclear factor-κB (NF-κB), interferon (IFN) response factors (IRFs), and mitogen-activated protein (MAP) kinases. These molecules induce the transcription of several pro-inflammatory molecules, such as interleukin (IL)-6, IL-8, IL-12, and tumor necrosis factor-α (TNF-α). AP1, activator protein 1; ATF, activating transcription factor; dsRNA, double-stranded RNA; ERK, extracellular signal-regulated kinase; IKK, inhibitor of kappa light polypeptide gene enhancer in B-cell kinase; IRAK, IL-1 receptor-associated kinase; JNK, c-Jun N-terminal kinase; LPS, lipopolysaccharide; MD, myeloid differentiation factor; MKK, MAPK kinase; NA, nucleic acid; TAB, transforming growth factor-β-activated kinase 1/MAP3K7-binding protein; TAK, transforming growth factor-activated kinase; TRAF, tumor necrosis factor receptor-associated factor; RIP1, receptor-interacting protein 1. Adapted from Anwar et al. [53].

http://dx.doi.org/10.5772/intechopen.80625

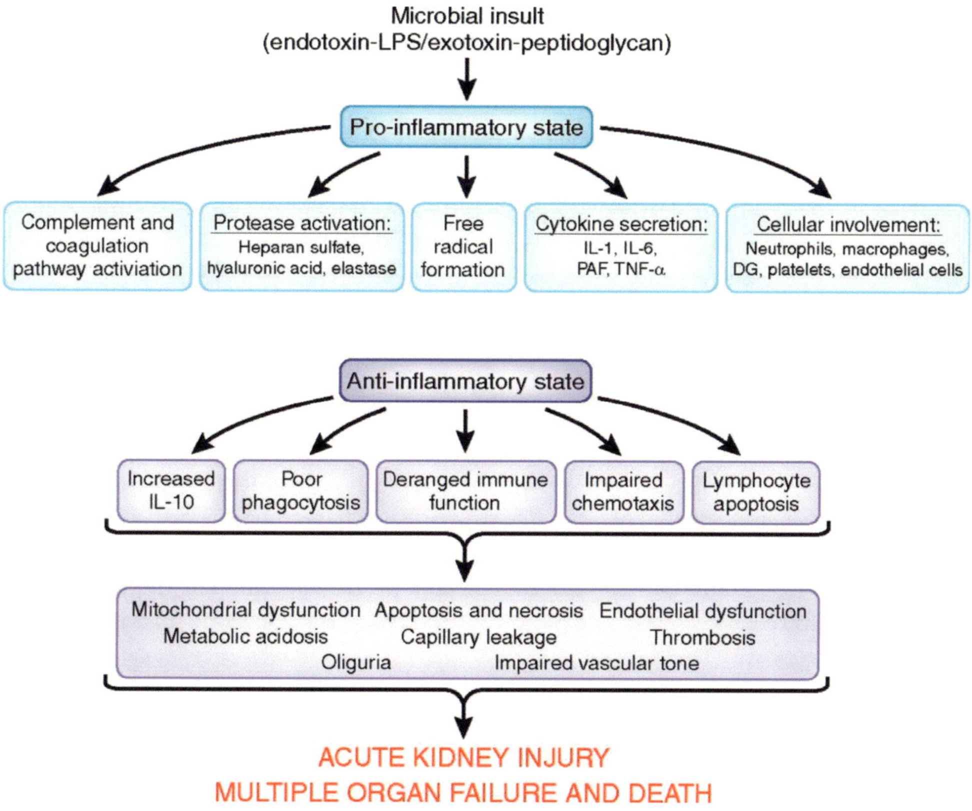

Figure 2. Key pathogenic pathways involved in sepsis that also have implications in the pathophysiology of sepsis-induced acute kidney injury. Adapted from Zarjou and Agarwal [42].

5. Clinical presentation of acute kidney injury

The clinical presentation of AKI depends on the cause and severity of renal insult. Mild to moderate AKI is asymptomatic and patients are identified based on laboratory testing. However, patients with severe AKI often present with a variety of symptoms including fatigue, anorexia, nausea, vomiting, restlessness, confusion, fluid retention, and weight gain. Severe and prolonged AKI may cause central nervous system manifestations such as uremic encephalopathy with asterixis, confusion, and seizure; bleeding tendency due to platelet dysfunction and severe anemia. Patients with AKI may have normal urine output, oliguria (urine output less than 400 mL/24 h) or anuria (urine output less than 100 mL/24 h).

6. Diagnosis of acute kidney injury

History and physical examination, with an emphasis on assessing the patient's volume status, are crucial for determining the cause of AKI. The history should inquire about the use of nephrotoxic medications or presence of systemic illnesses that might impair renal perfusion or directly impair renal function. Physical examination should assess the intravascular volume status and any skin rashes that indicate systemic diseases. The initial laboratory evaluation should include urinalysis, urine microscopy, complete blood count, electrolytes, serum creatinine or cystatin C level, and fractional excretion of sodium (FENa). Urinalysis and urine microscopy are essential in the initial work up of AKI. Findings on urinalysis and urine microscopy guide the differential diagnosis and direct further investigation. Imaging studies in particular ultrasonography can help in the initial work up of AKI. Ultrasonography is particularly important in older men with AKI who may have bladder outlet obstruction as a result of prostate hypertrophy [55, 56]. Renal biopsy is reserved for patients with AKI where the cause is not clear. Renal biopsy is particularly important when there is suspicion of an underlying disease that requires specific therapy such as glomerulonephritis or interstitial nephritis. Renal biopsy should be performed urgently in cases of rapidly progressive glomerulonephritis as indicated by rising serum creatinine or cystatin C and presence of red blood cell casts or dysmorphic red blood cells on urine microscopy.

7. New biomarkers for the quick detection of acute kidney injury

Although the RIFLE and AKIN criteria, based on serum creatinine and urine output, were a step forward in diagnosing AKI, a reliable tool to differentiate between true parenchymal and prerenal azotemia in clinical practice is still lacking [57]. Lately, several papers on the use of new urinary and serum biomarkers for the diagnosis and prognostication of AKI have been published with the hope that these biomarkers will lead to a new era of earlier diagnosis, better prognostication and treatment. Some of the studied biomarkers are listed in **Table 4**. Although these biomarkers may help to understand some of the biochemical and biological processes during AKI, their utility in preventing and treating AKI at present is at most very limited [58].

Acronym	Legend	Main source
AP	Alkaline phosphatase	Liver, bone, intestine, placenta, brush border proximal convoluted tubules
α_1MG	Alpha 1 microglobulin	Liver. Reabsorption by renal proximal tubular cells
$\alpha_1$acidGP	Alpha 1 acid glycoprotein	Liver. Reabsorption by renal proximal tubular cells
B_2MG	Beta 2 microglobulin	All nucleated cells. Reabsorption by renal proximal tubular cells
Cystatin C	Cystatin C	All nucleated cells. Reabsorption by renal proximal tubular cells
FENA	Fractional excretion of sodium	
GGTP	Gamma glutamyl transpeptidase	All cells except myocytes. Mainly liver and kidney (brush border proximal convoluted tubules and loop of Henle)

Acronym	Legend	Main source
αGST	Alpha-glutathione S-transferase	Expressed in almost all tissues. Kidney: proximal tubular cells (cytoplasmatic)
πGST	Pi glutathione S-transferase	Expressed in almost all tissues. Kidney: distal tubular cells (cytoplasmatic)
HGF	Hepatocyte growth factor	Mesenchymal cells
IL-6	Interleukin 6	T lymphocytes, macrophages, endothelial cells, monocytes
IL-8	Interleukin 8	Monocytes, macrophages, epithelial cells, endothelial cells
IL-10	Interleukin 10	Monocytes, lymphocytes, macrophages
IL-18	Interleukin 18	Monocytes, dendritic cells, macrophages and epithelial cells
KIM-1	Kidney injury molecule 1	Kidney: proximal tubular cells
LFABP	Liver-type fatty acid-binding protein	Hepatocytes, kidney: proximal tubular cells
NGAL	Neutrophil gelatinase-associated lipocalin	Leucocytes, loop of Henle and collecting ducts
NAG	*N*-Acetyl beta glucosaminidase	Several tissues (liver, brain, spleen, etc.). Kidney: proximal tubular cells (lysosomal)
PAI-1	Plasminogen activator inhibitor 1	Endothelium
PCX	Podocalyxin	Podocytes
RBP	Retinol-binding protein	Liver. Reabsorption by renal proximal tubular cells
sTNFR-I	Soluble tumor necrosis factor receptor I	Most cells and tissues (cytotoxic, apoptotic, and pro-inflammatory effects)
sTNFR-II	Soluble tumor necrosis factor receptor II	Most cells and tissues (proliferative and anti-apoptotic effects)
TNF-α	Tumor necrosis factor alpha	Macrophages, lymphoid cells, renal parenchymal cells
11 k-TXB_2	11-keto-Thromboxane B_2	Platelets
vWF	Von Willebrand factor	Endothelium, megakaryocytes, subendothelial connective tissue
TIMP-2	Tissue inhibitor of metalloproteinase-2	Ubiquitous expression. Renal tubular cells
IGFBP7	Insulin-like growth factor-binding protein 7	Ubiquitous expression. Renal tubular cells

Adapted and modified from Vanmassenhove [57].

Table 4. Urinary and serum biomarkers for the diagnosis of acute kidney injury.

8. Management of acute kidney injury

Management of AKI mandates close collaboration among nephrologists and other physicians involved in the care of the patient. The clinical evaluation of AKI includes a careful history and thorough physical examination. Drug history should include over-the-counter medications, herbal remedies, and recreational drugs [59]. Once established, management of AKI is mainly supportive. Most patients with AKI should be hospitalized unless the condition is mild and attributed to an easily reversible cause. The evaluation and initial management of patients with AKI should include: (1) an assessment of the contributing causes of the kidney injury, (2) an assessment of the clinical course including comorbidities, (3) a careful assessment of volume status, and (4) the institution of appropriate therapeutic measures designed to reverse or prevent worsening of functional or structural kidney abnormalities [60]. The initial assessment of patients with AKI should include the differentiation between prerenal, renal, and postrenal causes [34, 61–63]. In the majority of cases, the exclusion of postrenal causes using ultrasonography is an established approach and sufficient for the initial assessment. Differentiation between prerenal and renal causes is more challenging as renal hypoperfusion may coexist with any stage of AKI.

Assuring adequate renal perfusion by achieving and maintaining hemodynamic stability and avoiding hypovolemia is crucial in the initial management of AKI. Measurement of central venous pressures may be helpful in case of difficulty in assessing intravascular volume. Prerenal azotemia is rapidly reversible when the underlying cause is corrected [34, 60–63]. It is important to point out that certain elements of the definition of prerenal azotemia have diagnostic limitations. In the setting of renal hypoperfusion, compensatory mechanisms aimed at maintaining GFR may become operative. These compensatory mechanisms include efferent arteriolar vasoconstriction, afferent arteriolar dilation, and neuro/hormonal changes that lead to increased tubular reabsorption of solutes and water [64]. This implies that patients with renal hypoperfusion may be classified as having AKI by urine output criteria without having a significant change in serum creatinine concentration.

Volume resuscitation can correct prerenal conditions resulting from absolute or relative hypovolemia. However, renal hypoperfusion resulting from low cardiac output (severe cardiomyopathy) and reduced renal perfusion pressure (sepsis, or end-stage liver disease) cannot always be corrected by fluid administration [60]. Isotonic solutions (e.g., 0.9 sodium chloride) are preferred over hyperoncotic solutions due to the detrimental effect of these solutions (e.g., dextrans, hydroxyethyl starch, and albumin) [65, 66]. The use of hydroxyethyl starch as a plasma-volume expander has been shown to be an independent risk factor for AKI in patients with severe sepsis or septic shock [65]. In patients with persistent hypotension, vasopressors may be needed to maintain a mean blood pressure of 65 mmHg [66].

9. Pharmacologic interventions for management of acute kidney injury

A number of pharmacologic interventions have been evaluated in the early management of AKI. Some have been designed to improve renal perfusion and others to modulate intrarenal pathophysiology. In patients with hyperdynamic septic shock, both norepinephrine and terlipressin were effective in raising mean arterial blood pressure (MAP) leading to an improvement in renal function [67].

Low-dose (renal-dose) dopamine was frequently used in the ICU setting for its presumed renoprotective effects. Low-dose dopamine may increase the urine output on the first day of use, but prospective and retrospective studies as well as several meta-analyses have not shown positive effect in prevention of AKI or improvement in renal function in patients with AKI [68–71]. To the contrary, low-dose dopamine has been shown to worsen renal perfusion in patients with established AKI [72]. Therefore, the routine use of low-dose dopamine in critically ill patients should be abandoned.

Randomized controlled trials of early AKI and contrast nephropathy studying fenoldopam, a selective dopamine A1 agonist, proved this agent is ineffective at protecting renal function or reducing the need for renal replacement [73, 74]. Fenoldopam has been shown, however, to lower the risk of AKI in cardiac and major surgery patients according to some meta-analyses, without an effect on renal replacement or hospital mortality [75, 76]. In most of these studies, fenoldopam was associated with hypotension.

High-chloride fluids may be associated with increased risk of AKI and mortality in patients with sepsis [77]. Early goal-directed therapy with close monitoring of central venous pressure, mean arterial pressure, and oxygen saturation has been shown to be protective against AKI in patients admitted to the intensive care unit with sepsis [78, 79].

Atrial natriuretic peptide (ANP) is produced by cardiac atrial myocytes in response to atrial distension or increased atrial pressure. It induces afferent dilatation and efferent vasoconstriction, thereby increasing glomerular filtration and urinary sodium excretion [80]. B-type (brain) natriuretic peptide (BNP) is primarily produced in the cardiac ventricles and has similar effects [81, 82]. Low doses of recombinant human ANP-enhanced renal excretory function, decreased the probability of dialysis, and improved dialysis-free survival in early, ischemic acute renal dysfunction after complicated cardiac surgery [83]. Similar effects were observed in patients undergoing liver transplantation [84, 85]. However, larger doses of ANP were not effective in improving dialysis-free survival or reduction in dialysis in large randomized clinical trials [86, 87].

Theophylline, an adenosine antagonist has been shown in several preliminary reports to be beneficial in the prevention of contrast nephropathy and cisplatin nephrotoxicity [88–90]. A few adjunctive agents such as flavonoids (silymarin) and carotenoids (lycopene), have been tried in pilot studies in cancer patients receiving cisplatin with limited success in some but not all studies [91–93]. Adequately powered, controlled studies to support the efficacy of these agents are lacking.

Levosimendan, a calcium sensitizer, has inodilator, cardioprotective, and anti-inflammatory effects [94]. Two meta-analyses suggested that the use of levosimendan was associated with a reduction of renal replacement therapy in critically ill patients and patients undergoing cardiac surgery [95, 96]. The studies in both meta-analyses were small, heterogeneous, and AKI was not always a predefined endpoint.

The role of loop diuretics and osmotic agents in the prevention and treatment of AKI in humans has been disappointing despite their ability to decrease the tubular oxygen consumption and relieve intratubular obstruction in animal models [97–99]. A metanalysis has shown that frusemide was not associated with any significant clinical benefits in the prevention and treatment of AKI in adults, in addition to the concern of increased risk of ototoxicity associated with high doses [100].

N-acetyl-cysteine, a thiol-containing antioxidant has been investigated in several trials, mainly in the prevention of contrast-induced nephropathy. Despite some positive reports [101, 102], the protective effect of N-acetyl-cysteine is still controversial [103–106]. Similarly, N-acetyl-cysteine was not found to be protective against other causes of AKI particularly in hypotensive patients in the ICU or patients undergoing cardiac surgery [107, 108]. Hydration with sodium bicarbonate, as compared to normal saline, has been shown in some studies to be superior to normal saline in the prevention of contrast-induced nephropathy [109–111]. Other studies have shown no superiority of sodium bicarbonate over saline in the prevention of contrast nephropathy [112, 113]. Hydration with isotonic solutions either normal saline or sodium bicarbonate in addition to the use of low osmolar contrast agents is the most effective strategy to prevent contrast-induced nephropathy.

Statins may have a beneficial effect in high-risk patients exposed to contrast administration for angiography. In a randomized multicenter clinical trial, the short-term use of rosuvastatin was found to be protective against contrast nephropathy in diabetic patients with concomitant CKD who underwent coronary/peripheral arterial angiography [114]. In another single center trial high-dose rosuvastatin (40 mg on admission followed by 20 mg daily) given to statin-naïve patients with acute coronary syndrome who were scheduled for an early invasive procedure was protective against contrast-induced AKI and improved the short-term clinical outcome [115]. 6.7% of patients in the early high-dose rosuvastatin group developed AKI compared to 15.1% in the control group. The 30-day rate of adverse cardiovascular and renal events was also reduced in the rosuvastatin group (3.6 versus 7.9%). In a subgroup analysis of this study, rosuvastatin had a protective effect among female diabetic patients with CKD [116]. Similarly, a single high dose of atorvastatin (80 mg) administered within 24 h before exposure to intravenous contrast was effective in reducing the rate of AKI in diabetic patients with renal dysfunction [117, 118]. The protective effect of statins has been confirmed in multiple meta-analyses [119–121]. However, the beneficial effect of statins in patients undergoing coronary interventions was not observed in patients undergoing cardiac surgery. In this group of patients, the use of statin either showed no benefit or was detrimental [122–124].

10. Renal replacement therapy for acute kidney injury

There is a wide variation in clinical practice relating to the indication for and timing of RRT for patients with AKI. There is also no agreement on the selection of the specific modality of RRT and prescription of intensity of therapy. Among the several modalities of RRT, continuous renal replacement therapy has become very popular, especially in the ICU setting where patients may be hemodynamically unstable to tolerate intermittent hemodialysis. There does not appear to be a significant difference in either mortality or recovery of renal function associated with the various modalities of RRT. This is discussed in details in other sections of the book designated for RRT.

http://dx.doi.org/10.5772/intechopen.80625

11. Prevention of acute kidney injury

Acute kidney injury is particularly common in ICU patients affecting more than 50% and is associated with increased mortality and morbidity [16]. The Working Group on Prevention, AKI section, European Society of Intensive Care Medicine has recently issued recommendations for the prevention of AKI, specifically addressing the role of fluids, diuretics, inotropes, vasopressors/vasodilators, hormonal and nutritional interventions, sedatives, statins, remote ischemic preconditioning, and care bundles as shown in **Table 5** [125]. The recommendations are summarized as follows: timely resuscitation with fluids, vasopressors, and inotropic agents remains the cornerstone in the prevention of AKI. Volume expansion with isotonic crystalloids is reserved for true and suspected hypovolemia. The use of starches and dextrans should be avoided. In hypotensive patients, vasoconstrictors, preferably norepinephrine, should be administered with or following volume expansion. Mean arterial pressure (MAP) of 65–70 mmHg is adequate in most patients except in cases of preexisting chronic hypertension where a higher MAP (80–85 mmHg) should be targeted. Review of all medications and cessation of nephrotoxic agents is mandatory. Diuretics should not be used for prevention of AKI but may benefit in cases of volume overload and congestion. Hyperglycemia should be avoided. The effect of statins appears to depend on the setting, with promising results in contrast administration but no effect or even harm in cardiac surgery patients [125].

Volume expansion
Controlled fluid resuscitation in volume depletion, while, however, avoiding volume overload (1 C)
Avoidance of starches, gelatine, and dextrans (2C)
Correction of hypovolemia/dehydration using isotonic crystalloids in patients receiving intravascular contrast media (1 B)
Regular monitoring of chloride levels and acid–base status in situations where chloride-rich solutions are used (BPS)
Use of balanced crystalloids for large volume resuscitation (2C)
Use of human albumin if necessary for the treatment of patients with septic shock (2C).
Use of diuretics
No loop diuretics for the prevention of AKI (Grade 1B)
Diuretics to control or avoid fluid overload in patients that are diuretic-responsive (Grade 2D)
Use of vasopressors
Titrating vasopressors to a MAP of 65–70 mmHg (Grade 1B) in patients with septic shock and to (80–85 mmHg) for patients with chronic HTN (Grade 1C).
lowering SBP to 140–190 mmHg in patients with acute cerebral hemorrhage with severe admission hypertension (Grade 1C)
Norepinephrine as the first-choice vasopressor to protect kidney function (Grade 1B) and vasopressin in patients with vasoplegic shock after cardiac surgery (Grade 2C).
Individualizing target pressure when premorbid blood pressure is available (BPS)

Use of vasodilators

No low-dose dopamine for protection against AKI (Grade 1A)

No levosimendan for renal protection in patients with sepsis and in cardiac surgery patients with poor preoperative left ventricular function (Grade 1B).

No fenoldopam or natriuretic peptides for renal protection in critically ill or cardiovascular surgery patients at risk of AKI (Grade 2B).

Sedatives

Shorter sedation using propofol or dexmedetomidine (BPS)

Hormonal manipulation

Target a blood glucose level of at least below 180 mg/dL (10 mmol/l) (Grade 2B).

Use of erythropoietin or steroids (Grade 2 B)

Metabolic interventions

Avoid using high-dose IV selenium for renal protection in critically ill patients (1B)

Avoid using N-acetylcysteine to prevent contrast-associated AKI in critically ill patients (Grade 2B)

Provide adequate nutritional support preferably through the enteral route (BPS)

Statins

Avoid the use of high-dose statins to prevent postoperative AKI in cardiac surgery (Grade 1A)

Use atorvastatin or rosuvastatin to prevent contrast-associated AKI in high-risk patients undergoing coronary contrast angiography (Grade 2B)

Remote ischemic preconditioning

Do not use remote ischemic preconditioning for prevention of AKI in critically ill patients

AKI care bundles

Use of the KDIGO recommendations to reduce the incidence of AKI after cardiac surgery (Grade 2C).

Use of AKI care bundles outside the intensive care unit has some benefits, including the potential to improve the outcome of AKI (BPS).

AKI, acute kidney injury; HTN, hypertension; MAP, mean arterial pressure; BPS, best practice statement.

Table 5. Expert opinion of the Working Group on Prevention, AKI section, European Society of Intensive Care Medicine [125].

12. Prognosis of acute kidney injury

With the advent of agreed definition and classification of AKI based on changes in serum creatinine and urine output, there is now increasing awareness of the poor prognosis following AKI. Multiple studies have shown that patients with AKI are at high risk for progression to advanced stage CKD and death following hospital discharge. In a meta-analysis of 13 cohort studies comparing the risk of CKD, ESRD, and death in patients with and without AKI, the pooled incidence of CKD and ESRD were 25.8/100 person-years and 8.6/100 person-years, respectively [8]. Patients with AKI had higher risks of developing CKD (pooled adjusted hazard ratio 8.8), ESRD (pooled adjusted HR 3.1), and mortality (pooled adjusted HR 2.0) than patients without AKI [8]. In another meta-analysis of 48 studies containing 47,107 patients between 1985 and 2007 the incidence rate of mortality was 8.9 deaths/100 person-years in survivors of AKI compared to 4.3 deaths/100 patient-years in survivors without AKI (rate ratio 2.59) [126]. The incidence rate of CKD after an episode of AKI was 7.8 events/100 patient-years, and the rate of ESRD was 4.9 events/100 patient-years [126]. In an observational cohort study with a median follow-up of 9 years the intermediate-term (30–364 days) adjusted mortality HRs for AKI versus no AKI were 2.48, 2.50, 1.90, and 1.63 for baseline eGFRs ≥60, 45–59, 30–44, and <30 mL/min/1.73 m^2, respectively [127]. This indicates that baseline renal function is an important determinant factor for outcome following an episode of AKI. A retrospective cohort study showed that patients who developed AKI during a hospitalization were at substantial risk for the development of CKD in the following year, and the timing of recovery was a strong predictor, even for the mildest forms of AKI [128].

The multinational AKI-EPI study on ICU patients in 97 centers showed that increasing AKI severity was associated with increased mortality, and AKI patients had worse renal function at the time of hospital discharge [16].

According to the United States Renal Data System, acute tubular necrosis (ATN) without recovery as a cause of ESRD increased from 1.2% in 1994 to 1998 to 1.7% in 1999 to 2003 [129]. The incidence will likely continue to rise with the aging population and increase in comorbidities in patients admitted to the ICU.

Risk factors associated with progressing to CKD among AKI survivors have been identified and include advanced age, diabetes mellitus, decreased baseline glomerular filtration rate, severity of AKI, and a low concentration of serum albumin [6, 130].

13. Conclusion

Acute kidney injury, previously named acute renal failure, is characterized by abrupt deterioration in renal function. The incidence of AKI has lately increased, both in the hospital and community setting. Management of AKI involves fluid resuscitation, avoidance of nephrotoxic agents, adjustment of medications, and correction of fluid, acid-base and electrolyte imbalance. Depending on the severity of renal insult, AKI may require renal replacement therapy in the form of dialysis or continuous renal replacement. Despite all the advances in the field, AKI still carries a high mortality and long term consequences. Recognition of risk factors, early diagnosis, and management of AKI are crucial to improve the long-term patient's outcome.

Author details

Ahmed M. Alkhunaizi

Address all correspondence to: aalkhunaizi@gmail.com

Nephrology Section, Specialty Internal Medicine Unit, Johns Hopkins Aramco Healthcare, Dhahran, Saudi Arabia

References

[1] Mehta RL, Cerda J, Burdmann EA, Tonelli M, Garcia-Garcia G, Jha V, et al. International Society of Nephrology's 0by25 initiative for acute kidney injury (zero preventable deaths by 2025): A human rights case for nephrology. Lancet. 2015;**385**(9987):2616-2643

[2] Susantitaphong P, Cruz DN, Cerda J, Abulfaraj M, Alqahtani F, Koulouridis I, et al. World incidence of AKI: A meta-analysis. Clinical Journal of the American Society of Nephrology. 2013;**8**(9):1482-1493

[3] Silver SA, Chertow GM. The economic consequences of acute kidney injury. Nephron. 2017;**137**(4):297-301

[4] Cerda J, Bagga A, Kher V, Chakravarthi RM. The contrasting characteristics of acute kidney injury in developed and developing countries. Nature Clinical Practice. Nephrology. 2008;**4**(3):138-153

[5] Jha V, Parameswaran S. Community-acquired acute kidney injury in tropical countries. Nature Reviews. Nephrology. 2013;**9**(5):278-290

[6] Chawla LS, Eggers PW, Star RA, Kimmel PL. Acute kidney injury and chronic kidney disease as interconnected syndromes. The New England Journal of Medicine. 2014; **371**(1):58-66

[7] Ishani A, Xue JL, Himmelfarb J, Eggers PW, Kimmel PL, Molitoris BA, et al. Acute kidney injury increases risk of ESRD among elderly. Journal of the American Society of Nephrology. 2009;**20**(1):223-228

[8] Coca SG, Singanamala S, Parikh CR. Chronic kidney disease after acute kidney injury: A systematic review and meta-analysis. Kidney International. 2012;**81**(5):442-448

[9] Bedford M, Farmer C, Levin A, Ali T, Stevens P. Acute kidney injury and CKD: Chicken or egg? American Journal of Kidney Diseases. 2012;**59**(4):485-491

[10] Zuk A, Bonventre JV. Acute kidney injury. Annual Review of Medicine. 2016;**67**:293-307

[11] Lopes JA, Jorge S. The RIFLE and AKIN classifications for acute kidney injury: A critical and comprehensive review. Clinical Kidney Journal. 2013;**6**(1):8-14

[12] Bellomo R, Ronco C, Kellum JA, Mehta RL, Palevsky P. Acute renal failure—Definition, outcome measures, animal models, fluid therapy and information technology needs: The Second International Consensus Conference of the Acute Dialysis Quality Initiative [ADQI] Group. Critical Care. 2004;**8**(4):R204-R212

[13] Mehta RL, Kellum JA, Shah SV, Molitoris BA, Ronco C, Warnock DG, et al. Acute kidney injury network: Report of an initiative to improve outcomes in acute kidney injury. Critical Care. 2007;**11**(2):R31

[14] KDIGO. Improving global outcomes (KDIGO) Acute Kidney Injury Work Group. KDIGO clinical practice guideline for acute kidney injury. Kidney International. Supplement. 2012;**2**(1):S1-S138

[15] Rahman M, Shad F, Smith MC. Acute kidney injury: A guide to diagnosis and management. American Family Physician. 2012;**86**(7):631-639

[16] Hoste EA, Bagshaw SM, Bellomo R, Cely CM, Colman R, Cruz DN, et al. Epidemiology of acute kidney injury in critically ill patients: The multinational AKI-EPI study. Intensive Care Medicine. 2015;**41**(8):1411-1423

[17] Aksu U, Demirci C, Ince C. The pathogenesis of acute kidney injury and the toxic triangle of oxygen, reactive oxygen species and nitric oxide. Contributions to Nephrology. 2011; **174**:119-128

[18] Molitoris BA. Therapeutic translation in acute kidney injury: The epithelial/endothelial axis. The Journal of Clinical Investigation. 2014;**124**(6):2355-2363

[19] Ferenbach DA, Bonventre JV. Mechanisms of maladaptive repair after AKI leading to accelerated kidney ageing and CKD. Nature Reviews. Nephrology. 2015;**11**(5):264-276

[20] Basile DP, Donohoe D, Roethe K, Osborn JL. Renal ischemic injury results in permanent damage to peritubular capillaries and influences long-term function. American Journal of Physiology. Renal Physiology. 2001;**281**(5):F887-F899

[21] Inagi R. Endoplasmic reticulum stress in the kidney as a novel mediator of kidney injury. Nephron. Experimental Nephrology. 2009;**112**(1):e1-e9

[22] Zhang K, Kaufman RJ. From endoplasmic-reticulum stress to the inflammatory response. Nature. 2008;**454**(7203):455-462

[23] Raturi A, Simmen T. Where the endoplasmic reticulum and the mitochondrion tie the knot: The mitochondria-associated membrane [MAM]. Biochimica et Biophysica Acta. 2013;**1833**(1):213-224

[24] Venkatachalam MA, Griffin KA, Lan R, Geng H, Saikumar P, Bidani AK. Acute kidney injury: A springboard for progression in chronic kidney disease. American Journal of Physiology. Renal Physiology. 2010;**298**(5):F1078-F1094

[25] Brooks C, Wei Q, Cho SG, Dong Z. Regulation of mitochondrial dynamics in acute kidney injury in cell culture and rodent models. The Journal of Clinical Investigation. 2009;**119**(5):1275-1285

[26] Zhan M, Brooks C, Liu F, Sun L, Dong Z. Mitochondrial dynamics: Regulatory mechanisms and emerging role in renal pathophysiology. Kidney International. 2013;**83**(4):568-581

[27] Jiang M, Wei Q, Dong G, Komatsu M, Su Y, Dong Z. Autophagy in proximal tubules protects against acute kidney injury. Kidney International. 2012;**82**(12):1271-1283

[28] He L, Livingston MJ, Dong Z. Autophagy in acute kidney injury and repair. Nephron. Clinical Practice. 2014;**127**(1-4):56-60

[29] Kimura T, Isaka Y, Yoshimori T. Autophagy and kidney inflammation. Autophagy. 2017; **13**(6):997-1003

[30] Bonventre JV, Zuk A. Ischemic acute renal failure: An inflammatory disease? Kidney International. 2004;**66**(2):480-485

[31] Jang HR, Rabb H. Immune cells in experimental acute kidney injury. Nature Reviews. Nephrology. 2015;**11**(2):88-101

[32] Ysebaert DK, De Greef KE, Vercauteren SR, Ghielli M, Verpooten GA, Eyskens EJ, et al. Identification and kinetics of leukocytes after severe ischaemia/reperfusion renal injury. Nephrology, Dialysis, Transplantation. 2000;**15**(10):1562-1574

[33] Zuk A, Gershenovich M, Ivanova Y, MacFarland RT, Fricker SP, Ledbetter S. CXCR4 antagonism as a therapeutic approach to prevent acute kidney injury. American Journal of Physiology. Renal Physiology. 2014;**307**(7):F783-F797

[34] Schrier RW, Wang W, Poole B, Mitra A. Acute renal failure: Definitions, diagnosis, pathogenesis, and therapy. The Journal of Clinical Investigation. 2004;**114**(1):5-14

[35] Yu L, Gengaro PE, Niederberger M, Burke TJ, Schrier RW. Nitric oxide: A mediator in rat tubular hypoxia/reoxygenation injury. Proceedings of the National Academy of Sciences of the United States of America. 1994;**91**(5):1691-1695

[36] Noiri E, Peresleni T, Miller F, Goligorsky MS. In vivo targeting of inducible NO synthase with oligodeoxynucleotides protects rat kidney against ischemia. The Journal of Clinical Investigation. 1996;**97**(10):2377-2383

[37] Ling H, Gengaro PE, Edelstein CL, Martin PY, Wangsiripaisan A, Nemenoff R, et al. Effect of hypoxia on proximal tubules isolated from nitric oxide synthase knockout mice. Kidney International. 1998;**53**(6):1642-1646

[38] Kohjimoto Y, Kennington L, Scheid CR, Honeyman TW. Role of phospholipase A2 in the cytotoxic effects of oxalate in cultured renal epithelial cells. Kidney International. 1999; **56**(4):1432-1441

[39] Burke JE, Dennis EA. Phospholipase A2 biochemistry. Cardiovascular Drugs and Therapy. 2009;**23**(1):49-59

[40] Alkhunaizi AM, Yaqoob MM, Edelstein CL, Gengaro PE, Burke TJ, Nemenoff RA, et al. Arachidonic acid protects against hypoxic injury in rat proximal tubules. Kidney International. 1996;**49**(3):620-625

[41] Zager RA, Schimpf BA, Gmur DJ, Burke TJ. Phospholipase A2 activity can protect renal tubules from oxygen deprivation injury. Proceedings of the National Academy of Sciences of the United States of America. 1993;**90**(17):8297-8301

[42] Zarjou A, Agarwal A. Sepsis and acute kidney injury. Journal of the American Society of Nephrology. 2011;**22**(6):999-1006

[43] Lafrance JP, Miller DR. Acute kidney injury associates with increased long-term mortality. Journal of the American Society of Nephrology. 2010;**21**(2):345-352

[44] Bagshaw SM, Lapinsky S, Dial S, Arabi Y, Dodek P, Wood G, et al. Acute kidney injury in septic shock: Clinical outcomes and impact of duration of hypotension prior to initiation of antimicrobial therapy. Intensive Care Medicine. 2009;**35**(5):871-881

[45] Wan L, Bagshaw SM, Langenberg C, Saotome T, May C, Bellomo R. Pathophysiology of septic acute kidney injury: What do we really know? Critical Care Medicine. 2008;**36**(4 Suppl):S198-S203

[46] Devarajan P, Basu RK. Sepsis-associated acute kidney injury—Is it possible to move the needle against this syndrome? Jornal de Pediatria [Rio J]. 2017;**93**(1):1-3

[47] Hotchkiss RS, Karl IE. The pathophysiology and treatment of sepsis. The New England Journal of Medicine. 2003;**348**(2):138-150

[48] Martins PS, Brunialti MK, da Luz Fernandes M, Martos LS, Gomes NE, Rigato O, et al. Bacterial recognition and induced cell activation in sepsis. Endocrine, Metabolic & Immune Disorders Drug Targets. 2006;**6**(2):183-191

[49] Chow JC, Young DW, Golenbock DT, Christ WJ, Gusovsky F. Toll-like receptor-4 mediates lipopolysaccharide-induced signal transduction. The Journal of Biological Chemistry. 1999;**274**(16):10689-10692

[50] Kumar H, Kawai T, Akira S. Toll-like receptors and innate immunity. Biochemical and Biophysical Research Communications. 2009;**388**(4):621-625

[51] Armstrong L, Medford AR, Hunter KJ, Uppington KM, Millar AB. Differential expression of toll-like receptor [TLR]-2 and TLR-4 on monocytes in human sepsis. Clinical and Experimental Immunology. 2004;**136**(2):312-319

[52] Yang RB, Mark MR, Gray A, Huang A, Xie MH, Zhang M, et al. Toll-like receptor-2 mediates lipopolysaccharide-induced cellular signalling. Nature. 1998;**395**(6699):284-288

[53] Anwar MA, Basith S, Choi S. Negative regulatory approaches to the attenuation of toll-like receptor signaling. Experimental & Molecular Medicine. 2013;**45**:e11

[54] Atan R, Crosbie D, Bellomo R. Techniques of extracorporeal cytokine removal: A systematic review of the literature. Blood Purification. 2012;**33**(1-3):88-100

[55] O'Neill WC. Renal relevant radiology: Use of ultrasound in kidney disease and nephrology procedures. Clinical Journal of the American Society of Nephrology. 2014;**9**(2):373-381

[56] Gosmanova EO, Wu S, O'Neill WC. Application of ultrasound in nephrology practice. Advances in Chronic Kidney Disease. 2009;**16**(5):396-404

[57] Vanmassenhove J, Vanholder R, Nagler E, Van Biesen W. Urinary and serum biomarkers for the diagnosis of acute kidney injury: An in-depth review of the literature. Nephrology, Dialysis, Transplantation. 2013;**28**(2):254-273

[58] Lameire NH, Vanholder RC, Van Biesen WA. How to use biomarkers efficiently in acute kidney injury. Kidney International. 2011;**79**(10):1047-1050

[59] Kellum JA, Lameire N. Diagnosis, evaluation, and management of acute kidney injury: A KDIGO summary (Part 1). Critical Care. 2013;**17**(1):204

[60] Himmelfarb J, Joannidis M, Molitoris B, Schietz M, Okusa MD, Warnock D, et al. Evaluation and initial management of acute kidney injury. Clinical Journal of the American Society of Nephrology. 2008;**3**(4):962-967

[61] Thadhani R, Pascual M, Bonventre JV. Acute renal failure. The New England Journal of Medicine. 1996;**334**(22):1448-1460

[62] Fry AC, Farrington K. Management of acute renal failure. Postgraduate Medical Journal. 2006;**82**(964):106-116

[63] Lameire N, Van Biesen W, Vanholder R. Acute renal failure. Lancet. 2005;**365**(9457):417-430

[64] Badr KF, Ichikawa I. Prerenal failure: A deleterious shift from renal compensation to decompensation. The New England Journal of Medicine. 1988;**319**(10):623-629

[65] Schortgen F, Lacherade JC, Bruneel F, Cattaneo I, Hemery F, Lemaire F, et al. Effects of hydroxyethylstarch and gelatin on renal function in severe sepsis: A multicentre randomised study. Lancet. 2001;**357**(9260):911-916

[66] Brochard L, Abroug F, Brenner M, Broccard AF, Danner RL, Ferrer M, et al. An official ATS/ERS/ESICM/SCCM/SRLF statement: Prevention and management of acute renal failure in the ICU patient: An international consensus conference in intensive care medicine. American Journal of Respiratory and Critical Care Medicine. 2010;**181**(10): 1128-1155

[67] Albanese J, Leone M, Delmas A, Martin C. Terlipressin or norepinephrine in hyperdynamic septic shock: A prospective, randomized study. Critical Care Medicine. 2005; **33**(9):1897-1902

[68] Denton MD, Chertow GM, Brady HR. "Renal-dose" dopamine for the treatment of acute renal failure: Scientific rationale, experimental studies and clinical trials. Kidney International. 1996;**50**(1):4-14

[69] Friedrich JO, Adhikari N, Herridge MS, Beyene J. Meta-analysis: Low-dose dopamine increases urine output but does not prevent renal dysfunction or death. Annals of Internal Medicine. 2005;**142**(7):510-524

[70] Karthik S, Lisbon A. Low-dose dopamine in the intensive care unit. Seminars in Dialysis. 2006;**19**(6):465-471

[71] Holmes CL, Walley KR. Bad medicine: Low-dose dopamine in the ICU. Chest. 2003; **123**(4):1266-1275

[72] Lauschke A, Teichgraber UK, Frei U, Eckardt KU. 'Low-dose' dopamine worsens renal perfusion in patients with acute renal failure. Kidney International. 2006;**69**(9):1669-1674

[73] Tumlin JA, Finkel KW, Murray PT, Samuels J, Cotsonis G, Shaw AD. Fenoldopam mesylate in early acute tubular necrosis: A randomized, double-blind, placebo-controlled clinical trial. American Journal of Kidney Diseases. 2005;**46**(1):26-34

[74] Bove T, Zangrillo A, Guarracino F, Alvaro G, Persi B, Maglioni E, et al. Effect of fenoldopam on use of renal replacement therapy among patients with acute kidney injury after cardiac surgery: A randomized clinical trial. Journal of the American Medical Association. 2014;**312**(21):2244-2253

[75] Gillies MA, Kakar V, Parker RJ, Honore PM, Ostermann M. Fenoldopam to prevent acute kidney injury after major surgery-a systematic review and meta-analysis. Critical Care. 2015;**19**:449

[76] Zangrillo A, Biondi-Zoccai GG, Frati E, Covello RD, Cabrini L, Guarracino F, et al. Fenoldopam and acute renal failure in cardiac surgery: A meta-analysis of randomized placebo-controlled trials. Journal of Cardiothoracic and Vascular Anesthesia. 2012;**26**(3): 407-413

[77] Jaynes MP, Murphy CV, Ali N, Krautwater A, Lehman A, Doepker BA. Association between chloride content of intravenous fluids and acute kidney injury in critically ill medical patients with sepsis. Journal of Critical Care. 2018;**44**:363-367

[78] Rivers E, Nguyen B, Havstad S, Ressler J, Muzzin A, Knoblich B, et al. Early goal-directed therapy in the treatment of severe sepsis and septic shock. The New England Journal of Medicine. 2001;**345**(19):1368-1377

[79] Stone GW, McCullough PA, Tumlin JA, Lepor NE, Madyoon H, Murray P, et al. Fenoldopam mesylate for the prevention of contrast-induced nephropathy: A randomized controlled trial. Journal of the American Medical Association. 2003;**290**(17): 2284-2291

[80] Sward K, Valsson F, Sellgren J, Ricksten SE. Differential effects of human atrial natriuretic peptide and furosemide on glomerular filtration rate and renal oxygen consumption in humans. Intensive Care Medicine. 2005;**31**(1):79-85

[81] Kuhn M. Endothelial actions of atrial and B-type natriuretic peptides. British Journal of Pharmacology. 2012;**166**(2):522-531

[82] Kuhn M. The natriuretic peptide/guanylyl cyclase—A system functions as a stress-responsive regulator of angiogenesis in mice. Journal of Clinical Investigation. 2009;**119** (7):2019-2030

[83] Sward K, Valsson F, Odencrants P, Samuelsson O, Ricksten SE. Recombinant human atrial natriuretic peptide in ischemic acute renal failure: A randomized placebo-controlled trial. Critical Care Medicine. 2004;**32**(6):1310-1315

[84] Akamatsu N, Sugawara Y, Tamura S, Kaneko J, Togashi J, Kishi Y, et al. Prevention of renal impairment by continuous infusion of human atrial natriuretic peptide after liver transplantation. Transplantation. 2005;**80**(8):1093-1098

[85] Sato K, Sekiguchi S, Kawagishi N, Akamatsu Y, Enomoto Y, Takeda I, et al. Continuous low-dose human atrial natriuretic peptide promotes diuresis in oliguric patients after living donor liver transplantation. Transplantation Proceedings. 2006;**38**(10):3591-3593

[86] Allgren RL, Marbury TC, Rahman SN, Weisberg LS, Fenves AZ, Lafayette RA, et al. Anaritide in acute tubular necrosis. Auriculin Anaritide Acute Renal Failure Study Group. The New England Journal of Medicine. 1997;**336**(12):828-834

[87] Lewis J, Salem MM, Chertow GM, Weisberg LS, McGrew F, Marbury TC, et al. Atrial natriuretic factor in oliguric acute renal failure. Anaritide Acute Renal Failure Study Group. American Journal of Kidney Diseases. 2000;**36**(4):767-774

[88] Bagshaw SM, Ghali WA. Theophylline for prevention of contrast-induced nephropathy: A systematic review and meta-analysis. Archives of Internal Medicine. 2005;**165**(10): 1087-1093

[89] Ix JH, McCulloch CE, Chertow GM. Theophylline for the prevention of radiocontrast nephropathy: A meta-analysis. Nephrology, Dialysis, Transplantation. 2004;**19**(11): 2747-2753

[90] Benoehr P, Krueth P, Bokemeyer C, Grenz A, Osswald H, Hartmann JT. Nephroprotection by theophylline in patients with cisplatin chemotherapy: A randomized, single-blinded, placebo-controlled trial. Journal of the American Society of Nephrology. 2005;**16**(2):452-458

[91] Momeni A, Hajigholami A, Geshnizjani S, Kheiri S. Effect of silymarin in the prevention of Cisplatin nephrotoxicity, a clinical trial study. Journal of Clinical and Diagnostic Research. 2015;**9**(4):OC11-OC13

[92] Shahbazi F, Sadighi S, Dashti-Khavidaki S, Shahi F, Mirzania M, Abdollahi A, et al. Effect of silymarin administration on cisplatin nephrotoxicity: Report from a pilot, randomized, double-blinded, placebo-controlled clinical trial. Phytotherapy Research. 2015;**29**(7): 1046-1053

[93] Mahmoodnia L, Mohammadi K, Masumi R. Ameliorative effect of lycopene effect on cisplatin-induced nephropathy in patient. Journal of Nephropathology. 2017;**6**(3):144-149

[94] Hasslacher J, Bijuklic K, Bertocchi C, Kountchev J, Bellmann R, Dunzendorfer S, et al. Levosimendan inhibits release of reactive oxygen species in polymorphonuclear leukocytes in vitro and in patients with acute heart failure and septic shock: A prospective observational study. Critical Care. 2011;**15**(4):R166

[95] Bove T, Matteazzi A, Belletti A, Paternoster G, Saleh O, Taddeo D, et al. Beneficial impact of levosimendan in critically ill patients with or at risk for acute renal failure: A meta-analysis of randomized clinical trials. Heart Lung Vessel. 2015;**7**(1):35-46

[96] Zhou C, Gong J, Chen D, Wang W, Liu M, Liu B. Levosimendan for prevention of acute kidney injury after cardiac surgery: A meta-analysis of randomized controlled trials. American Journal of Kidney Diseases. 2016;**67**(3):408-416

[97] Brezis M, Agmon Y, Epstein FH. Determinants of intrarenal oxygenation. I. Effects of diuretics. The American Journal of Physiology. 1994;**267**(6 Pt 2):F1059-F1062

[98] Mehta RL, Pascual MT, Soroko S, Chertow GM. Diuretics, mortality, and nonrecovery of renal function in acute renal failure. Journal of the American Medical Association. 2002; **288**(20):2547-2553

[99] Solomon R, Werner C, Mann D, D'Elia J, Silva P. Effects of saline, mannitol, and furosemide on acute decreases in renal function induced by radiocontrast agents. The New England Journal of Medicine. 1994;**331**(21):1416-1420

[100] Ho KM, Sheridan DJ. Meta-analysis of frusemide to prevent or treat acute renal failure. BMJ. 2006;**333**(7565):420

[101] Tepel M, van der Giet M, Schwarzfeld C, Laufer U, Liermann D, Zidek W. Prevention of radiographic-contrast-agent-induced reductions in renal function by acetylcysteine. The New England Journal of Medicine. 2000;**343**(3):180-184

[102] Marenzi G, Assanelli E, Marana I, Lauri G, Campodonico J, Grazi M, et al. N-acetylcysteine and contrast-induced nephropathy in primary angioplasty. The New England Journal of Medicine. 2006;**354**(26):2773-2782

[103] Bagshaw SM, McAlister FA, Manns BJ, Ghali WA. Acetylcysteine in the prevention of contrast-induced nephropathy: A case study of the pitfalls in the evolution of evidence. Archives of Internal Medicine. 2006;**166**(2):161-166

[104] Kama A, Yilmaz S, Yaka E, Dervisoglu E, Dogan NO, Erimsah E, et al. Comparison of short-term infusion regimens of N-acetylcysteine plus intravenous fluids, sodium bicarbonate plus intravenous fluids, and intravenous fluids alone for prevention of contrast-induced nephropathy in the emergency department. Academic Emergency Medicine. 2014;**21**(6):615-622

[105] Traub SJ, Mitchell AM, Jones AE, Tang A, O'Connor J, Nelson T, et al. N-acetylcysteine plus intravenous fluids versus intravenous fluids alone to prevent contrast-induced nephropathy in emergency computed tomography. Annals of Emergency Medicine. 2013;**62**(5):511-520. e25

[106] Hynninen MS, Niemi TT, Poyhia R, Raininko EI, Salmenpera MT, Lepantalo MJ, et al. N-acetylcysteine for the prevention of kidney injury in abdominal aortic surgery: A randomized, double-blind, placebo-controlled trial. Anesthesia and Analgesia. 2006;**102**(6): 1638-1645

[107] Komisarof JA, Gilkey GM, Peters DM, Koudelka CW, Meyer MM, Smith SM. N-acetylcysteine for patients with prolonged hypotension as prophylaxis for acute renal failure [NEPHRON]. Critical Care Medicine. 2007;**35**(2):435-441

[108] Nigwekar SU, Kandula P. N-acetylcysteine in cardiovascular-surgery-associated renal failure: A meta-analysis. The Annals of Thoracic Surgery. 2009;**87**(1):139-147

[109] Merten GJ, Burgess WP, Gray LV, Holleman JH, Roush TS, Kowalchuk GJ, et al. Prevention of contrast-induced nephropathy with sodium bicarbonate: A randomized controlled trial. Journal of the American Medical Association. 2004;**291**(19):2328-2334

[110] Briguori C, Airoldi F, D'Andrea D, Bonizzoni E, Morici N, Focaccio A, et al. Renal Insufficiency Following Contrast Media Administration Trial [REMEDIAL]: A randomized comparison of 3 preventive strategies. Circulation. 2007;**115**(10):1211-1217

[111] Ozcan EE, Guneri S, Akdeniz B, Akyildiz IZ, Senaslan O, Baris N, et al. Sodium bicarbonate, N-acetylcysteine, and saline for prevention of radiocontrast-induced nephropathy. A comparison of 3 regimens for protecting contrast-induced nephropathy in patients undergoing coronary procedures. A single-center prospective controlled trial. American Heart Journal. 2007;**154**(3):539-544

[112] Maioli M, Toso A, Leoncini M, Gallopin M, Tedeschi D, Micheletti C, et al. Sodium bicarbonate versus saline for the prevention of contrast-induced nephropathy in patients with renal dysfunction undergoing coronary angiography or intervention. Journal of the American College of Cardiology. 2008;**52**(8):599-604

[113] Schmidt P, Pang D, Nykamp D, Knowlton G, Jia H. N-acetylcysteine and sodium bicarbonate versus N-acetylcysteine and standard hydration for the prevention of radiocontrast-induced nephropathy following coronary angiography. The Annals of Pharmacotherapy. 2007;**41**(1):46-50

[114] Han Y, Zhu G, Han L, Hou F, Huang W, Liu H, et al. Short-term rosuvastatin therapy for prevention of contrast-induced acute kidney injury in patients with diabetes and chronic kidney disease. Journal of the American College of Cardiology. 2014;**63**(1):62-70

[115] Leoncini M, Toso A, Maioli M, Tropeano F, Villani S, Bellandi F. Early high-dose rosuvastatin for contrast-induced nephropathy prevention in acute coronary syndrome: Results from the PRATO-ACS study [Protective effect of rosuvastatin and antiplatelet therapy on contrast-induced acute kidney injury and myocardial damage in patients with acute coronary syndrome]. Journal of the American College of Cardiology. 2014;**63**(1):71-79

[116] Li J, Li Y, Xu B, Jia G, Guo T, Wang D, et al. Short-term rosuvastatin therapy prevents contrast-induced acute kidney injury in female patients with diabetes and chronic kidney disease: A subgroup analysis of the TRACK-D study. Journal of Thoracic Disease. 2016; **8**(5):1000-1006

[117] Quintavalle C, Fiore D, De Micco F, Visconti G, Focaccio A, Golia B, et al. Impact of a high loading dose of atorvastatin on contrast-induced acute kidney injury. Circulation. 2012; **126**(25):3008-3016

[118] Shehata M, Hamza M. Impact of high loading dose of atorvastatin in diabetic patients with renal dysfunction undergoing elective percutaneous coronary intervention: A randomized controlled trial. Cardiovascular Therapeutics. 2015;**33**(2):35-41

[119] Barbieri L, Verdoia M, Schaffer A, Nardin M, Marino P, De Luca G. The role of statins in the prevention of contrast induced nephropathy: A meta-analysis of 8 randomized trials. Journal of Thrombosis and Thrombolysis. 2014;**38**(4):493-502

[120] Lee JM, Park J, Jeon KH, Jung JH, Lee SE, Han JK, et al. Efficacy of short-term high-dose statin pretreatment in prevention of contrast-induced acute kidney injury: Updated study-level meta-analysis of 13 randomized controlled trials. PLoS One. 2014;**9**(11):e111397

[121] Ukaigwe A, Karmacharya P, Mahmood M, Pathak R, Aryal MR, Jalota L, et al. Meta-analysis on efficacy of statins for prevention of contrast-induced acute kidney injury in patients undergoing coronary angiography. The American Journal of Cardiology. 2014;**114**(9):1295-1302

[122] Billings FT, Hendricks PA, Schildcrout JS, Shi Y, Petracek MR, Byrne JG, et al. High-dose perioperative atorvastatin and acute kidney injury following cardiac surgery: A randomized clinical trial. Journal of the American Medical Association. 2016;**315**(9):877-888

[123] Park JH, Shim JK, Song JW, Soh S, Kwak YL. Effect of atorvastatin on the incidence of acute kidney injury following valvular heart surgery: A randomized, placebo-controlled trial. Intensive Care Medicine. 2016;**42**(9):1398-1407

[124] Zheng Z, Jayaram R, Jiang L, Emberson J, Zhao Y, Li Q, et al. Perioperative rosuvastatin in cardiac surgery. The New England Journal of Medicine. 2016;**374**(18):1744-1753

[125] Joannidis M, Druml W, Forni LG, Groeneveld ABJ, Honore PM, Hoste E, et al. Prevention of acute kidney injury and protection of renal function in the intensive care unit: Update 2017: Expert opinion of the Working Group on Prevention, AKI section, European Society of Intensive Care Medicine. Intensive Care Medicine. 2017;**43**(6):730-749

[126] Coca SG, Yusuf B, Shlipak MG, Garg AX, Parikh CR. Long-term risk of mortality and other adverse outcomes after acute kidney injury: A systematic review and meta-analysis. American Journal of Kidney Diseases. 2009;**53**(6):961-973

[127] Sawhney S, Marks A, Fluck N, Levin A, Prescott G, Black C. Intermediate and long-term outcomes of survivors of acute kidney injury episodes: A large population-based cohort study. American Journal of Kidney Diseases. 2017;**69**(1):18-28

[128] Heung M, Steffick DE, Zivin K, Gillespie BW, Banerjee T, Hsu CY, et al. Acute kidney injury recovery pattern and subsequent risk of CKD: An analysis of veterans health administration data. American Journal of Kidney Diseases. 2016;**67**(5):742-752

[129] Goldberg R, Dennen P. Long-term outcomes of acute kidney injury. Advances in Chronic Kidney Disease. 2008;**15**(3):297-307

[130] Chawla LS. Acute kidney injury leading to chronic kidney disease and long-term outcomes of acute kidney injury: The best opportunity to mitigate acute kidney injury? Contributions to Nephrology. 2011;**174**:182-190

Chapter 3

Hemodiafiltration in Acute Kidney Injury

Kullaya Takkavatakarn,
Paweena Susantitaphong and Somchai Eiam-Ong

Additional information is available at the end of the chapter

http://dx.doi.org/10.5772/intechopen.79563

Abstract

Acute kidney injury (AKI) is one of the most important complications during hospitalization, especially in critically ill patients. Recent data demonstrated that certain biomarkers including pro-inflammatory cytokines are associated with high morbidity and mortality. These biomarkers, most of which have middle molecular weight, and protein-bound uremic toxins are limitedly removed by diffusion mechanism in conventional hemodialysis. Hemodiafiltration (HDF), a new modality that combines convective clearance with diffusion, could effectively enhance removal of middle molecule and protein-bound solutes. Therefore, HDF is increasingly used in several AKI settings such as septic AKI, rhabdomyolysis-associated AKI, myeloma cast nephropathy, and contrast-induced AKI. This chapter summarizes the available HDF techniques including intermittent and continuous modes, and clinical data comprise the benefits of HDF on biomarkers and renal as well as cardiovascular outcomes. Additionally, the topic provides the proposed future directions of HDF in various AKI settings.

Keywords: acute kidney injury, hemodiafiltration, convection, diffusion, sepsis, rhabdomyolysis, myeloma

1. Background

Acute kidney injury (AKI) is one of the most serious complications of patients during hospitalization especially in critically ill patients [1]. The annual incidence and mortality of AKI have been escalating despite much improvement of patient cares [2]. Besides correcting the underlying causes of AKI, there is no specific medication for effective treatment of AKI. Nowadays, the main treatment of AKI is still limited to supportive management. However, some patients had refractory volume overload and severe metabolic derangement;

therefore, renal replacement therapy (RRT) has become a key management in patients with AKI and multi-organ failure in order to normalize fluid, electrolyte, and acid–base status. Hemodiafiltration (HDF), one of the recently innovative RRT modalities, could provide benefits in decreasing inflammatory markers and cytokines, which play an important role in various AKI entities.

2. Principles of renal replacement therapy (RRT)

There are two main transportation processes of solutes and fluid across a membrane during RRT, diffusion and convection [3].

2.1. Diffusion

Diffusion is the process of spontaneous migration of solutes from a higher concentration to a lower concentration across the semipermeable membrane until the concentration becomes equal throughout a space (**Figure 1**). Factors affecting diffusion are concentration gradients, molecular size and charge of the solutes, surface area, thickness, and solute permeability of the membrane. Diffusion is the main determinant mechanism of small solute clearance in hemodialysis (HD).

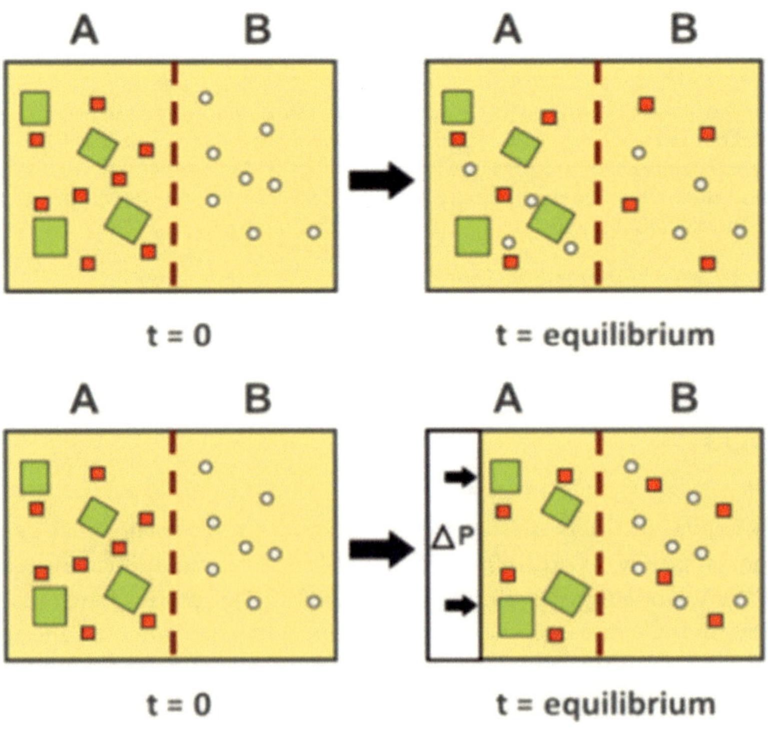

Figure 1. The processes of diffusion (top) and convection (bottom): O = Small solutes; ■ = Middle molecule and protein-bound solutes; ■ = Large solutes.

2.2. Convection (solvent drag)

Convection is the transportation process which the solutes migrate along with water flow (solvent) across the semipermeable membrane (**Figure 1**). Water flow or ultrafiltration is the movement of fluid across the membrane produced by transmembrane pressure gradients. There are many factors affecting the convection such as solute concentration gradients, sieving coefficient, surface area, pore size, and the permeability of membrane, but the most important one is ultrafiltration rate. Convection is able to remove protein-bound uremic toxins and middle molecule solutes such as interleukins, complement, platelet-activating factors, and other cytokines. This process is the main determinant mechanism of solute clearance in hemofiltration (HF).

3. HDF techniques

HDF is an RRT modality which combines diffusion and convection techniques to enhance the removal of middle molecule solutes and protein-bound uremic toxins by using high-flux dialyzer [4]. Therefore, this technique requires not only dialysate fluid but also sterile substitution fluid for replacement. There are various types of dilutional methods according to the site of replacement fluid infusion pre-dilution, post-dilution, mid-dilution, and mixed-dilution.

3.1. Pre-dilution HDF

In pre-dilution HDF, the replacement fluid is infused before the dialyzer (**Figure 2A**). Pre-dilution infusion reduces hemoconcentration across the membrane leading to prolongation of the extracorporeal circuit duration. However, this method provides less efficiency of solute clearance by diffusion.

3.2. Post-dilution HDF

Post-dilution HDF is the most efficient solute removal method of HDF due to high concentration gradient between blood and dialysate fluid. In post-dilution method, the replacement fluid is infused downstream the dialyzer (**Figure 2B**). An important disadvantage is that the increased hemoconcentration during high ultrafiltration rates would result in clogging of the membrane pores. Occlusion of the dialyzer leads to high transmembrane pressure gradient, reducing solute clearance, and, eventually, membrane leakage or clotting in the dialyzer.

3.3. Mid-dilution HDF

The replacement fluid is infused between two high-flux dialyzers placed in series resulting in a first post-dilution hemodiafiltration stage followed by a pre-dilution hemodiafiltration stage (**Figure 2C**). This technique can combine the advantage of both pre-dilution and post-dilution. However, the high transmembrane pressure and clotting in the first part of dialyzer are the important limitation of this technique.

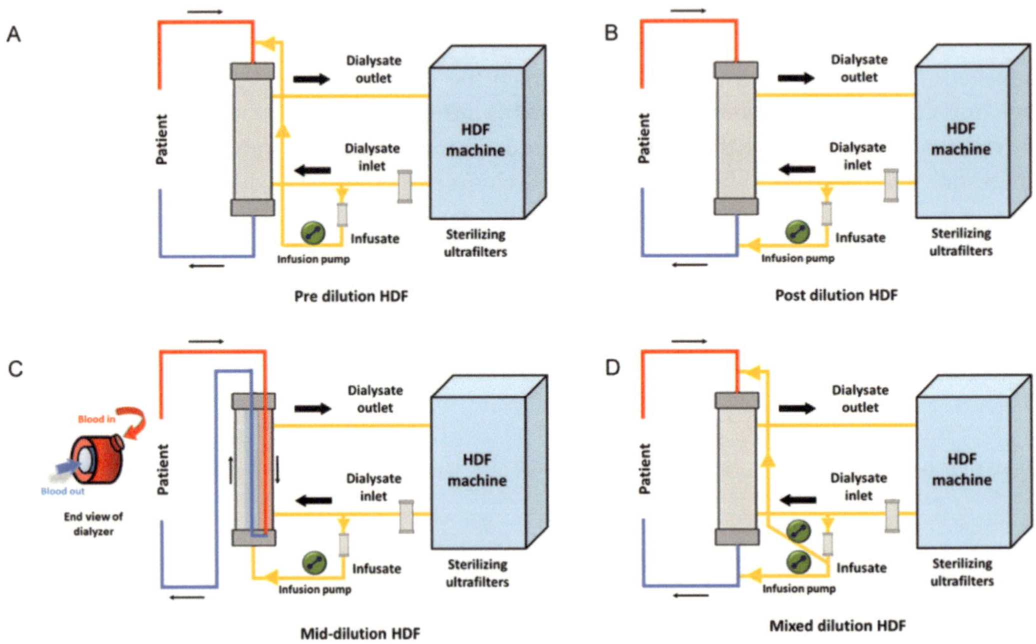

Figure 2. HDF modes according to the site of replacement fluid infusion: pre-dilution (A), post-dilution (B), mid-dilution (C), and mixed-dilution (D).

3.4. Mixed-dilution HDF

The replacement fluid is infused both before and after the dialyzer (**Figure 2D**). To reduce the unfavorable components of pre- and post-dilution HDF, the ratio of upstream and downstream infusion rates can be adjusted to achieve the optimal balance between maximizing clearance and avoiding hemoconcentration.

Of note, the efficacy of convection transport mainly depends on convection volume which consists of replacement fluid and ultrafiltration fluid. The classic HDF technique requires approximately 10 L of replacement fluid per session, while high-volume HDF uses at least 15 L per session for greater convection transport. Online HDF (OL-HDF) has been developed to reduce the high cost of commercial replacement fluid. OL-HDF is a technique using the dialysis fluid itself as the replacement fluid. After multiple steps of water purification process, the dialysis fluid becomes ultrapure before the final filtration and the last ultrafilter must have the capacity to create sterile substitutional fluid. This technique contributes a very high fluid turnover of 25–30 L per session and significantly improves middle molecule solute clearance [5, 6].

In summary, HDF has higher potency of removal of middle molecule solutes and protein-bound uremic toxins than the conventional HD [7]. Therefore, HDF would provide more benefits than conventional HD in patients with AKI particularly in certain situations, such as sepsis, rhabdomyolysis, and myeloma cast nephropathy, which requires more middle molecule solute clearance.

4. HDF and sepsis-induced AKI

Sepsis is the most common cause of AKI in critically ill patients. A line of evidence shows that AKI may occur in the absence of overt hemodynamic instability. The novel concepts in the pathophysiology of sepsis-induced AKI are explained by several mechanisms, including inflammation, alteration of microcirculatory flow, and cellular responses to the inflammatory insults (**Figure 3**) [8, 9].

Firstly, the pro-inflammatory cytokines produced in sepsis such as tumor necrosis factor (TNF), interleukin-1 (IL-1), interleukin-6 (IL-6), and interferon (IFN) could contribute direct renal tubular injury [10]. In addition to the large amount of pro-inflammatory cytokines, nitric oxide and vascular endothelial growth factor (VEGF) generated during sepsis are responsible for the distortion of renal microcirculation and endothelial dysfunction [11], even with normal or increased global renal blood flow [12]. These alterations provide heterogeneity of regional blood flow distribution, impair renal autoregulation, and finally promote renal dysfunction [13, 14]. At the cellular level, mitochondria is the common target of inflammatory injury, which leads to its dysfunction, increased production of reactive oxygen species (ROS), and cell cycle arrest [15, 16].

According to these mechanisms, hemodynamic compromise does not seem to be very significant to deteriorate renal function. A previous study demonstrated that hypotension does not correlate with AKI in patients with severe sepsis [17]. Meanwhile, the production of cytokines, nitric oxide, and ROS may be the key pathogenesis of sepsis-induced AKI. Moreover, prolonged release of inflammatory mediators leads to severely impaired immunity which is followed by the secondary infection [18]. Therefore, this immunoparalysis state plays an important role in the mortality of patients with sepsis. Restoration of immune homeostasis might be able to improve the outcomes [19].

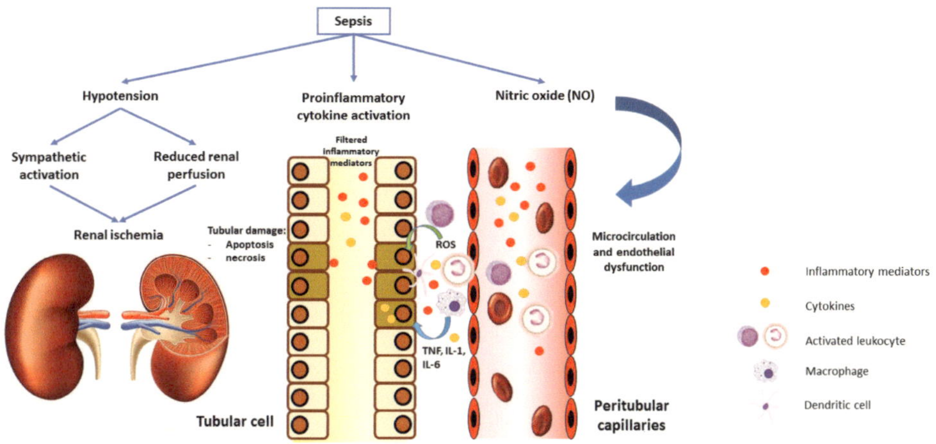

Figure 3. Pathophysiology of sepsis-induced AKI. Abbreviation: ROS, reactive oxygen species; TNF, tumor necrosis factor; IL-1, interleukin-1; IL-6, interleukin-6.

Theoretically, HDF could provide significantly higher middle molecule clearance including pro-inflammatory cytokines when compared with conventional HD. Therefore, many studies have tried to determine the benefits of HDF in sepsis-induced AKI. Indeed, a number of theories trying to explain the effects of blood purification have been proposed. First, Ronco et al. postulated that eliminating the peaks of cytokine concentration from the blood circulation during the early phase of sepsis could stop the inflammatory cascade, limit organ damage, and consequently decrease multi-organ failure [20]. The second concept is called "threshold immunomodulation hypothesis." Honore et al. proposed that cytokine removal affects not only the cytokine concentrations in bloodstream but also the level in tissues [21]. This is caused by an equilibration of their concentrations between the two compartments. According to this hypothesis, cytokines for the tissues replace those removed from the blood. Hence, no significant reduction in bloodstream cytokine concentration is observed during blood purification. The third concept is about immunomodulation. During blood purification therapy, the inflammatory cell could restore the immune function through the regulation of monocytes, neutrophils, and lymphocytes [22]. HF and HDF could play a role at this point by reducing a large amount of cytokines, terminating the inflammatory cascade, and promoting the immune recovery. However, the benefits of these modalities have been demonstrated in only limited studies.

There have been several observational studies in critically ill patients with multiple organ failure demonstrating that high-volume HF (HVHF) which prescribed at least 35 mL/kg/hr. of ultrafiltration volume or intermittent HDF improved patients' clinical outcomes [23–27]. Kron et al. performed an extended daily online high-volume HDF (6–23 hours) with convective volume about 173 L/treatment in patients with sepsis [28]. In this study, hemodynamics improved significantly during the treatment, and the 90-day survival rate compared with the survival rate predicted by severity scores (APACHE II and SAPS II) was 52 versus 19%. A previous prospective randomized controlled trial (RCT) in sepsis-induced AKI patients illustrated that pre-dilution intermittent OL-HDF for 4 hours enhanced cytokine removal over intermittent high-flux HD [29]. The clearance and reduction ratio of either pro-inflammatory or anti-inflammatory cytokines such as IL-6 (26 kDa), IL-8 (8 kDa), IL-10 (40 kDa), VEGF (46 kDa), and TNF-a (51 kDa) was significantly greater in OL-HDF than high-flux HD modality. Moreover, OL-HDF showed some better clinical outcomes including renal recovery and shorter length of hospital stay. Nevertheless, there was no significant difference in mortality between these two modalities. Another RCT, which compared every day or every alternate day of intermittent high-volume pre-dilution OL-HDF (the mean volume of replacement fluid is 81 L) to standard intermittent HD for 4 hours in critically ill ICU patients with AKI as part of multiple organ failure, failed to demonstrate the significant difference in mortality and kidney function recovery [30].

Most of critically ill patients with septic shock or hemodynamic instability require continuous RRT (CRRT). In addition to the advantage in maintaining hemodynamic stability through slow continuous ultrafiltration, many studies have proposed its ability in removal of pro-inflammatory cytokines and other middle molecule solutes through convection. Both continuous venovenous hemodiafiltration (CVVHDF) and continuous venovenous hemofiltration (CVVH) could be performed to increase convective transport. A retrospective, longitudinal follow-up study for 12 months in severe sepsis with AKI patients who received CRRT including CVVH and CVVHDF aiming at the dose of dialysis more than 35 mL/kg/hr. in ICU was performed [31]. There was no significant difference in survival rate between sepsis-induced

AKI patients treated with CVVH and CVVHDF. However, subgroup analysis in patients with oliguria/anuria showed significantly higher survival in patients treated with CVVHDF compared with CVVH. However, this result could actually be explained by the effect of residual renal clearance. In patients who still preserved diuresis, some pro-inflammatory cytokines were removed from plasma into the urine. Therefore, different CRRT modes might not affect the clinical outcomes. On the other hand, after loss of renal function, a large number of cytokines were more rapidly accumulated. A combination of diffusion and convection by CVVHDF might better control the cytokines and other uremic toxin accumulations and provided better survival outcome. However, this hypothesis needs further investigations.

4.1. Dose prescription

Besides the modalities of CRRT, the CRRT dose utilized for sepsis-induced AKI is still unestablished. Prescribed and delivered doses of CRRT in AKI vary widely. Two large, multicenter RCTs were conducted in critically ill patients with AKI to investigate the effects of RRT dose on survival benefit. The US Department of Veterans Affairs/National Institutes of Health conducted Acute Renal Failure Trial Network (ATN) study by randomly assigning 1124 critically ill patients with AKI who required RRT to high-intensity RRT (35 mL/kg/hr. of pre-dilution CVVHDF or six sessions per week of SLEDD/IHD) or low-intensity RRT (20 mL/kg/hr. of pre-dilutional CVVHDF or three sessions per week of SLEDD/IHD) [32]. The results showed survival rates after 60 days of 46% in high-intensity group and 48% in low-intensity group (p value = 0.47). In another RCT trial, the Randomized Evaluation of Normal versus Augmented Level (RENAL) of Replacement Therapy study of 1508 critically ill patients meeting the criteria for initiation RRT was included and randomly assigned to post-dilution CVVHDF with effluent rate of 40 or 25 mL/kg/hr [33]. There was no statistically significant difference of 90-day mortality between high- and low-dose RRT groups. Moreover, the secondary outcomes such as length of ICU and hospital stay, duration of mechanical ventilation therapy, and dialysis status at 90 days were not different. Both studies failed to demonstrate any benefits of using high-intensity RRT. Although the higher doses of CRRT are expected to provide more effective inflammatory cytokine removal in sepsis, subgroup analysis of patients with sepsis or organ failure revealed no significant differences in the mortality between the high- and low-intensity RRT. In addition, a recent prospective study in sepsis-induced AKI patients failed to demonstrate improvement in clinical outcomes of the high-dose pre-dilution CVVHDF over the conventional dose (80 vs. 40 mL/kg/hr) despite significant influence of high-dose CVVHDF in removal of IL-6, IL-8, and IL-10 [34]. Therefore, the KDIGO guidelines [35] proposed the optimal dose of CRRT of 20–25 mL/kg/hr in patients with AKI regardless of the etiologies of AKI. The studies examining the effects of RRT dose and outcomes are summarized in **Table 1**. However, delivering of the prescribed dose may be compromised due to filter clotting, concentration polarization of the filter, and other factors including access-related problems which diminish the treatment time. Rolando et al. studied the actual delivered dose of RRT in critically ill patients with AKI requiring dialysis. The delivered clearance was derived from the ratio of mass removal rate to blood concentration and effluent volume rate. From this study, the prescribed clearance overestimated the actual delivered clearance by 23.8% [36]. Therefore, the effluent rate prescription should be increased by 20–25% to achieve an actual prescribed dose.

Author/study	Type	Sample	Comparison/intervention	Outcomes
Comparing HDF and other modalities				
Dario et al. [23]	Multicenter, prospective, and comparative study	65 patients with AKI and sepsis	OL-HDF versus low-intensity high-flux IHD	OL-HDF showed benefits statistically significant in intensive care unit stay
Chancharoenthana et al. [29]	Single-center RCT	28 patients with AKI and sepsis	OL-HDF versus high-flux IHD	OL-HDF showed significant higher inflammatory cytokine removal, better renal recovery, and shorter length of hospital stay
Skofic et al. [30]	Single-center RCT	273 critically ill patients with AKI	High-volume OL-HDF (mean volume 81 L) versus standard IHD	No significant difference of mortality
Premuzic et al. [31]	Retrospective, longitudinal follow-up study for 12 months duration	137 patients with AKI and sepsis	CVVHDF versus CVVH aiming at the dose of dialysis >35 mL/kg/hr	No significant difference in survival rate Subgroup analysis in patients with oliguria/anuria showed significantly higher survival in patients treated with CVVHDF compared with CVVH
Effect of HDF dose and outcomes				
Kron et al. [28]	Prospective observational study	21 patients with AKI and sepsis	Extended daily online high-volume HDF (6–23 hours) with convective volume about 173 L/treatment in patients with sepsis	Significantly lower predicted mortality by APACHEII and SAPSII scores
ATN trial [32]	Multicenter RCT	1124 critically ill patients with AKI	Pre-dilution CVVHDF 35 ml/kg/r or six sessions/week of SLEDD/IHD versus pre-dilution CVVHDF 20 ml/kg/hr or three sessions/week of SLEDD/IHD	No significant difference of survival rate (46 and 48%)
RENAL trial [33]	Multicenter RCT	1508 critically ill patients with AKI	Post-dilution CVVHDF 40 ml/kg/hr versus 25 ml/kg/hr	No significant difference of survival rate (55 and 55%)
Park et al. [34]	Single-center RCT	212 patients with AKI and sepsis	High-dose pre-dilution CVVHDF 80 mL/kg/hr versus conventional dose pre-dilution CVVHDF 40 mL/kg/hr	Significant influence of high-dose CVVHDF in removal of inflammatory cytokines No significant difference of mortality

Table 1. Clinical trials using HDF in critically ill patients with AKI.

http://dx.doi.org/10.5772/intechopen.79563

5. HDF and rhabdomyolysis-induced AKI

Myoglobin is an oxygen-binding protein found in cardiac and skeletal muscle. It has a molecular mass of 17.9 kDa. In patients with normal renal function, a rapid rise in blood myoglobin levels would be followed by a rapid disappearance within 6 hours due to high renal clearance. Myoglobin clearance decreases in renal impairment and myoglobin elimination half-life could be extended to 21 hours (range 17–29 hours) in dialyzed patients [37].

In rhabdomyolysis, myoglobin, released from injured muscle into circulation, induces renal vasoconstriction, oxidative stress, direct tubular injury, and tubular obstruction. Besides promoting urine and renal clearance of myoglobin, effective removal by extracorporeal therapies might reduce renal injuries [38]. High-flux membranes typically allow clearance of molecules up to 20 kDa, while high cutoff (HCO) membranes permit molecules with 20–50 kDa. Some larger molecules such as albumin (65 kDa) and clotting factors may also be removed when convection is applied in HCO.

There was a case series reporting on HDF with a HCO membrane applied in the treatment of acute myoglobinuric renal failure [39]. Highly efficient myoglobin removal was demonstrated. By measuring myoglobin content in the collected effluent, the single HCO-HDF for 12 hours resulted in nearly 5 grams of myoglobin removal, with a mean myoglobin clearance of 80.7 mL/min. However, a high rebound in serum myoglobin on average to 244% of the post-procedure myoglobin level was observed. Several studies also reported mass myoglobin removal on CVVHF with high-flux or HCO membranes [40–43]. However, there was no strong evidence displaying the effects of myoglobin removal on renal recovery and mortality outcome in myoglobinuric renal failure patients.

6. HDF and myeloma cast nephropathy

AKI in patients with multiple myeloma is mostly related to myeloma cast nephropathy characterized by monoclonal light chain and uromodulin obstructions in distal tubules of the kidney. Cast nephropathy is generated by massive light chain secretion in the tubules and precipitated with reduction of tubular flow. There was an RCT comparing between intensive HD (eight 5-hour sessions over 10 days) with a HCO dialyzer (HCO-HD) and conventional HD among patients who were newly diagnosed with myeloma cast nephropathy and treated with a bortezomib-based chemotherapy regimen [44]. HCO-HD allowed higher clearance of both kappa (κ) and lambda (λ) light chains. Moreover, a rapid reduction of circulating monoclonal light chains by intensive HCO-HD resulted in a statistically significant difference in HD independence at 6 and 12 months (56.5 vs. 35.4%; $p = 0.04$ and 60.9 vs. 37.5%; $p = 0.02$, respectively). However, the HD-independent rate at 3 months which was the primary outcome was not significantly different. Although using HCO membrane was likely to improve the renal outcome, higher albumin loss during HCO-HD should be considered.

Regarding HDF, there was a case series demonstrating the efficacy of supra-hemodiafiltration with endogenous reinfusion (supra-HFR) which is a subtype of HDF that utilizes separated convection, diffusion, and adsorption [45]. The sorbent cartridge has a high affinity for both κ and λ free light chains without the drawback of albumin loss. In this report, more than 50% reduction of the serum free light chain levels occurred within only 1 week of supra-HFR treatment, and three out of four cases became dialysis independent after 2–6 weeks with no significant loss of albumin.

7. HDF and contrast-induced nephropathy (CIN)

CIN is a common cause of AKI which can range from a minor or transient elevation of serum creatinine to severe renal failure requiring dialysis. These injuries are associated with significant inhospital and long-term morbidity and mortality [46, 47]. Although various strategies in preventing CIN, such as acetylcysteine, theophylline, and other renoprotective drugs, have been evaluated, only intravenous administration of normal saline and sodium bicarbonate seem to be a useful method [48, 49].

Prophylactic HD starting immediately after administration of the contrast in patients with previous renal dysfunction failed to demonstrate the benefit in CIN prevention [50]. Nevertheless, Marenzi et al. reported the efficacy and safety of periprocedural CVVHF in chronic kidney disease patients undergoing coronary interventions (4–6 hours before coronary procedure and continued for 18–24 hours) [51]. The explanation for the discrepancy is that HD might induce hypovolemia, leading to renal hypoperfusion and renal ischemia which are important risk factors of CIN. On the contrary, CVVHF is corresponding with enhanced hemodynamic stability. In addition, CVVHF provides controlled high-volume hydration and could remove more contrast agent from the circulation, resulting in reduction of kidney exposure to the contrast agent. There was a study which compared the contrast media removing the ability of different extracorporeal treatments as low-flux HD, high-flux HD, HF, and HDF [52]. In this study, HDF and high-flux HD could effectively remove contrast media more effectively than low-flux HD and HF.

Katoh et al. performed HDF with blood suction from the right atrium (RA-HDF) in patients with renal dysfunction undergoing coronary angiography (CAG) or percutaneous coronary intervention (PCI) [53]. RA-HDF was started 30 minutes before the scheduled coronary procedure and continued until 30 minutes after the procedure. By this method, the blood was drawn from the right atrium near the orifice of the coronary sinus. Therefore, the contrast media injected into a coronary artery could be removed effectively before entering the systemic circulation. Although there was no statistically significant difference, the frequency of CI-AKI was lower in the patients receiving normal saline hydration in combination with RA-HDF compared with those administered only normal saline (12 vs. 27%). Another study investigated the use of prophylactic HDF for 3 hours after emergency or urgent CAG in acute coronary syndrome patients with severe renal (eGFR <30 mL/min/1.73 m^2) and cardiac dysfunctions (LVEF < 40%) [54]. Patients who were dialyzed with HDF had a lower incidence of severe AKI (10 vs. 40%) and lower requirement for RRT during hospitalization (7 vs. 27%). Moreover, they experienced significantly lower 1-year mortality rates than the controls. Taken together, prophylactic HDF is likely to provide salutary benefit in patients with very high risks who are undergoing coronary interventions. However, certain limitations should be considered. First, these reports are prospective observational studies with quite small number of patients. Second, prophylactic HDF is associated with high expense, and the cost-effectiveness should be evaluated. **Table 2** details the comparison of outcomes between HDF and conventional HD in various AKI entities.

Etiology of AKI	HDF vs. conventional HD
Sepsis-induced AKI	Significantly higher cytokine removal than HD
Cytokine removal	Probable benefits
Renal recovery	No benefit
Mortality	
Rhabdomyolysis	Significantly higher myoglobin removal
	No evidence of renal recovery and mortality benefit
Myeloma cast nephropathy	Significantly higher free light chain removal
	No evidence of renal recovery and mortality benefit
Prophylaxis of contrast-induced nephropathy	Periprocedure HDF reduce incidence if CIN

Abbreviations: AKI: acute kidney injury; HDF: hemodiafiltration; HD: hemodialysis; CIN-AKI: contrast-induced nephropathy-acute kidney injury.

Table 2. Comparison of outcomes between HDF and conventional HD in various AKI settings.

8. Conclusion

By combining diffusive and convective clearances, HDF is one of the most effective modalities in clearance of middle molecule solutes and protein-bound uremic toxins. In addition to the benefit of conventional uremic toxin clearance, HDF provides a significantly higher elimination of other nephrotoxic substances. This clearance capacity seems to be associated with the improvement of renal recovery and clinical outcomes in some special entities of AKI such as sepsis, rhabdomyolysis, myeloma cast nephropathy, and CIN. However, the reduction in the mortality of patients undergoing HDF is quite difficult to be evaluated. In conclusion, while there is rising of clinical evidence favoring HDF in AKI, further large-scale prospective RCTS are essentially required to confirm its benefits.

Author details

Kullaya Takkavatakarn, Paweena Susantitaphong and Somchai Eiam-Ong*

*Address all correspondence to: somchai80754@yahoo.com

Division of Nephrology, Department of Medicine, Faculty of Medicine, Chulalongkorn University, King Chulalongkorn Memorial Hospital, Bangkok, Thailand

References

[1] Singbartl K, Kellum JA. AKI in the ICU: Definition, epidemiology, risk stratification, and outcomes. Kidney International. 2012;**81**:819-825

[2] Zeng X, McMahon GM, Brunelli SM, Bates DW, Waikar SS. Incidence, outcomes, and comparisons across definitions of AKI in hospitalized individuals. Clinical Journal of the American Society of Nephrology. 2014;**9**:12-20

[3] Denisov A. The basic principles of blood purification during hemodialysis. Terapevticheskiĭ Arkhiv. 1996;**68**:69-74

[4] Ronco C, Cruz D. Hemodiafiltration history, technology, and clinical results. Advances in Chronic Kidney Disease. 2007;**14**:231-243

[5] Tattersall JE, Ward RA, Group E. Online haemodiafiltration: Definition, dose quantification and safety revisited. Nephrology, Dialysis, Transplantation. 2013;**28**:542-550

[6] Ledebo I. On-line preparation of solutions for dialysis: Practical aspects versus safety and regulations. Journal of the American Society of Nephrology. 2002;**13**(suppl 1):S78-S83

[7] Vanholder R, Meert N, Schepers E, Glorieux G. From uremic toxin retention to removal by convection: Do we know enough? Contributions to Nephrology. 2008;**161**:125-131

[8] Gomez H, Kellum J. Sepsis-induced acute kidney injury. Current Opinion in Critical Care. 2016;**22**:546-553

[9] De Backer D, Creteur J, Preiser J, Dubois M, Vincent J. Microvascular blood flow is altered in patients with sepsis. American Journal of Respiratory and Critical Care Medicine. 2002;**166**:98-104

[10] Bonventre JV, Yang L. Cellular pathophysiology of ischemic acute kidney injury. The Journal of Clinical Investigation. 2011;**121**:4210-4221

[11] Jean-Baptiste E. Cellular mechanisms in sepsis. Journal of Intensive Care Medicine. 2007;**22**:63-72

[12] Bezemer R, Legrand M, Klijn E, Heger M, Post IC, van Gulik TM, et al. Real-time assessment of renal cortical microvascular perfusion heterogeneities using near-infrared laser speckle imaging. Optics Express. 2010;**18**:15054-15061

[13] Verma S, Molitoris B. Renal endothelial injury and microvascular dysfunction in acute kidney injury. Seminars in Nephrology. 2015;**35**:96-107

[14] Tiwari M, Brock R, Megyesi J, Kaushal G, Mayeux P. Disruption of renal peritubular blood flow in lipopolysaccharide-induced renal failure: Role of nitric oxide and caspases. American Journal of Physiology. Renal Physiology. 2005;**289**:F1324-F1332

[15] Vanhorebeek I, Gunst J, Derde S, Derese I, Boussemaere M, D'Hoore A, et al. Mitochondrial fusion, fission, and biogenesis in prolonged critically ill patients. The Journal of Clinical Endocrinology and Metabolism. 2012;**97**:E59-E64

[16] Yang QH, Liu DW, Long Y, Liu HZ, Chai WZ, Wang XT. Acute renal failure during sepsis: Potential role of cell cycle regulation. The Journal of Infection. 2009;**58**:459-464

[17] Chawla LS, Seneff MG, Nelson DR, Williams M, Levy H, Kimmel PL, et al. Elevated plasma concentrations of IL-6 and elevated APACHE II score predict acute kidney injury in patients with severe sepsis. Clinical Journal of the American Society of Nephrology. 2007;**2**:22-30

[18] Hotchkiss RS, Coopersmith CM, McDunn JE, Ferguson TA. The sepsis seesaw: Tilting toward immunosuppression. Nature Medicine. 2009;**15**:496-497

[19] Hotchkiss RS, Karl IE. The pathophysiology and treatment of sepsis. The New England Journal of Medicine. 2003;**348**:138-150

[20] Ronco C, Tetta C, Mariano F, Wratten ML, Bonello M, Bordoni V, et al. Interpreting the mechanisms of continuous renal replacement therapy in sepsis: The peak concentration hypothesis. Artificial Organs. 2003;**27**:792-801

[21] Honoré PM, Matson JR. Extracorporeal removal for sepsis: Acting at the tissue level--the beginning of a new era for this treatment modality in septic shock. Critical Care Medicine. 2004;**32**:896-897

[22] Peng Z, Singbartl K, Simon P, Rimmele T, Bishop J, Clermont G, et al. Blood purification in sepsis: A new paradigm. Contributions to Nephrology. 2010;**165**:322-328

[23] Daríoe J, Manuel G, Ana A, Miguel M, Fernando J, et al. Intermittent hemodialysis low intensity vs. on line hemodiafiltration in critically ill patients with sepsis and acute kidney injury. Choosing the best treatment in a developing country. Journal of Nephrology and Therapeutics. 2017;**7**:299

[24] Cole L, Bellomo R, Journois D, Davenport P, Baldwin I, Tipping P. High-volume haemofiltration in human septic shock. Intensive Care Medicine. 2001;**27**:978-986

[25] Cornejo R, Downey P, Castro R, Romero C, Regueira T, Vega J, et al. High-volume hemofiltration as salvage therapy in severe hyperdynamic septic shock. Intensive Care Medicine. 2006;**32**:713-722

[26] Boussekey N, Chiche A, Faure K, Devos P, Guery B, d'Escrivan T, et al. A pilot randomized study comparing high and low volume hemofiltration on vasopressor use in septic shock. Intensive Care Medicine. 2008;**34**:1646-1653

[27] Honore PM, Jamez J, Wauthier M, Lee PA, Dugernier T, Pirenne B, et al. Prospective evaluation of short-term, high-volume isovolemic hemofiltration on the hemodynamic course and outcome in patients with intractable circulatory failure resulting from septic shock. Critical Care Medicine. 2000;**28**:3581-3587

[28] Kron J, Kron S, Wenkel R, Schuhmacher HU, Thieme U, Leimbach T, et al. Extended daily on-line high-volume haemodiafiltration in septic multiple organ failure: A well-tolerated and feasible procedure. Nephrology, Dialysis, Transplantation. 2012;**27**:146-152

[29] Chancharoenthana W, Tiranathanagul K, Srisawat N, Susantitaphong P, Leelahavanichkul A, Praditpornsilpa K, et al. Enhanced vascular endothelial growth factor and inflammatory cytokine removal with online hemodiafiltration over high-flux hemodialysis in sepsis-related acute kidney injury patients. Therapeutic Apheresis and Dialysis. 2013;**17**:557-563

[30] Skofic N, Arnol M, Buturovic-Ponikvar J, Ponikvar R. Intermittent high-volume predilution on-line haemofiltration versus standard intermittent haemodialysis in critically ill patients with acute kidney injury: A prospective randomized study. Nephrology, Dialysis, Transplantation. 2012;**27**:4348-4356

[31] Premuzic V, Basic-Jukic N, Jelakovic B, Kes P. Differences in CVVH vs. CVVHDF in the management of sepsis-induced acute kidney injury in critically ill patients. Journal of Artificial Organs. 2017;**20**:326-334

[32] Network VNARFT, Palevsky PM, Zhang JH, O'Connor TZ, Chertow GM, Crowley ST, et al. Intensity of renal support in critically ill patients with acute kidney injury. The New England Journal of Medicine. 2008;**359**:7-20

[33] Investigators RRTS, Bellomo R, Cass A, Cole L, Finfer S, Gallagher M, et al. Intensity of continuous renal-replacement therapy in critically ill patients. The New England Journal of Medicine. 2009;**361**:1627-1638

[34] Park JT, Lee H, Kee YK, Park S, Oh HJ, Han SH, et al. High-dose versus conventional-dose continuous venovenous hemodiafiltration and patient and kidney survival and cytokine removal in sepsis-associated acute kidney injury: A randomized controlled trial. American Journal of Kidney Diseases. 2016;**68**:599-608

[35] Kidney disease: Improving global outcomes (KDIGO) acute kidney injury work group KDIGO clinical practice guideline for acute kidney injury. Kidney International. Supplement. 2012;**2**:1-138

[36] Claure-Del Granado R, Macedo E, Chertow GM, Soroko S, Himmelfarb J, Ikizler TA, et al. Effluent volume in continuous renal replacement therapy overestimates the delivered dose of dialysis. Clinical Journal of the American Society of Nephrology. 2011;**6**:467-475

[37] Mikkelsen TS, Toft P. Prognostic value, kinetics and effect of CVVHDF on serum of the myoglobin and creatine kinase in critically ill patients with rhabdomyolysis. Acta Anaesthesiologica Scandinavica. 2005;**49**:859-864

[38] Bosch X, Poch E, Grau JM. Rhabdomyolysis and acute kidney injury. The New England Journal of Medicine. 2009;**361**:62-72

[39] Premru V, Kovac J, Buturovic-Ponikvar J, Ponikvar R. High cut-off membrane hemodiafiltration in myoglobinuric acute renal failure: A case series. Therapeutic Apheresis and Dialysis. 2011;**15**:287-291

[40] Bastani B, Frenchie D. Significant myoglobin removal during continuous veno-venous haemofiltration using F80 membrane. Nephrology, Dialysis, Transplantation. 1997;**12**: 2035-2036

[41] Amyot SL, LeBlanc M, Thibeault Y, Geadah D, Cardinal J. Myoglobin clearance and removal during continuous venovenous hemofiltration. Intensive Care Medicine. 1999;**25**:1169-1172

[42] Hutchison CA, Harding S, Basnayake K, B radwell AR, Cockwell P. Myoglobin removal by high cut-off hemodialysis: In-vivo studies. Journal of the American Society of Nephrology. 2007;**18**:250A

[43] Naka T, Jones D, Baldwin I, Fealy N, Bates S, Goehl H, et al. Myoglobin clearance by super high-flux hemofiltration in a case of severe rhabdomyolysis: A case report. Critical Care. 2005;**9**:R90-R95

[44] Bridoux F, Carron PL, Pegourie B, Alamartine E, Augeul-Meunier K, Karras A, et al. Effect of high-cutoff hemodialysis vs conventional hemodialysis on hemodialysis independence among patients with myeloma cast nephropathy: A randomized clinical trial. Journal of the American Medical Association. 2017;**318**:2099-2110

[45] Pasquali S, Iannuzzella F, Corradini M, Mattei S, Bovino A, Stefani A, et al. A novel option for reducing free light chains in myeloma kidney: Supra-hemodiafiltration with endogenous reinfusion (HFR). Journal of Nephrology. 2015;**28**(2):251-254

[46] Weisbord S, Palevsky P. Radiocontrast-induced acute renal failure. Journal of Intensive Care Medicine. 2005;**20**:63-75

[47] Weisbord SD, Mor MK, Resnick AL, Hartwig KC, Palevsky PM, Fine MJ. Incidence and outcomes of contrast-induced AKI following computed tomography. Clinical Journal of the American Society of Nephrology. 2008;**3**:1274-1281

[48] Mueller C, Buerkle G, Buettner HJ, Petersen J, Perruchoud AP, Eriksson U, et al. Prevention of contrast media-associated nephropathy: Randomized comparison of 2 hydration regimens in 1620 patients undergoing coronary angioplasty. Archives of Internal Medicine. 2002;**162**:329-336

[49] Zhang B, Liang L, Chen W, Liang C, Zhang S. The efficacy of sodium bicarbonate in preventing contrast-induced nephropathy in patients with pre-existing renal insufficiency: A meta-analysis. BMJ Open. 2015;**5**:e006989

[50] Vogt B, Ferrari P, Schonholzer C, Marti HP, Mohaupt M, Wiederkehr M, et al. Prophylactic hemodialysis after radiocontrast media in patients with renal insufficiency is potentially harmful. The American Journal of Medicine. 2001;**111**:692-698

[51] Marenzi G, Marana I, Lauri G, Assanelli E, Grazi M, Campodonico J, et al. The prevention of radiocontrast-agent-induced nephropathy by hemofiltration. The New England Journal of Medicine. 2003;**349**:1333-1340

[52] Schindler R, Stahl C, Venz S, Ludat K, Krause W, Frei U. Removal of contrast media by different extracorporeal treatments. Nephrology, Dialysis, Transplantation. 2001;**16**:1471-1474

[53] Katoh H, Nozue T, Kimura Y, Nakata S, Iwaki T, Kawano M, et al. Elevation of urinary liver-type fatty acid-binding protein as predicting factor for occurrence of contrast-induced acute kidney injury and its reduction by hemodiafiltration with blood suction from right atrium. Heart and Vessels. 2014;**29**:191-197

[54] Marenzi G, Mazzotta G, Londrino F, Gistri R, Moltrasio M, Cabiati A, et al. Post-procedural hemodiafiltration in acute coronary syndrome patients with associated renal and cardiac dysfunction undergoing urgent and emergency coronary angiography. Catheterization and Cardiovascular Interventions. 2015;**85**:345-351

Chapter 4

Immunoadsorption Techniques and Its Current Role in the Intensive Care Unit

Patrick Hamilton, Rhodri Harris and Sandip Mitra

Additional information is available at the end of the chapter

http://dx.doi.org/10.5772/intechopen.84890

Abstract

Immunoadsorption is an extracorporeal technique used for the removal of antibodies and molecules from the blood. A large number of different adsorbents are now available allowing for the non-selective removal of all subclasses of immunoglobulins such as IgG or more selective removal of disease specific molecules such as lipoprotein(a) and CRP. This selectivity, coupled with its highly efficient removal of the molecule, along with a favourable side-effect profile, has made immunoadsorption an attractive option in a range of autoimmune diseases. Here we discuss the mechanism and technique of immunoadsorption and review the current evidence and indications for its use, particularly in relation to sepsis.

Keywords: sepsis, immunoadsorption, extracorporeal therapy, autoimmune disease

1. Introduction

Immunoadsorption (IA) was developed in the 1990s as a method of extracorporeal removal of molecules from the blood, in particular molecules of the immune system. There are now a large number of devices/columns on the market, each with a different active component to which the molecule of interest attaches, allowing for selectivity in the molecules removed. This selectivity is one of immunoadsorption's significant advantages over other apheresis techniques, in that it negates the need for replacement of factors such as albumin and plasma. With the vast majority of IA systems directed against components of the immune system, its use has traditionally been in autoimmune conditions and transplantation, although new systems are increasingly being used for other indications such as sepsis (**Figure 1**).

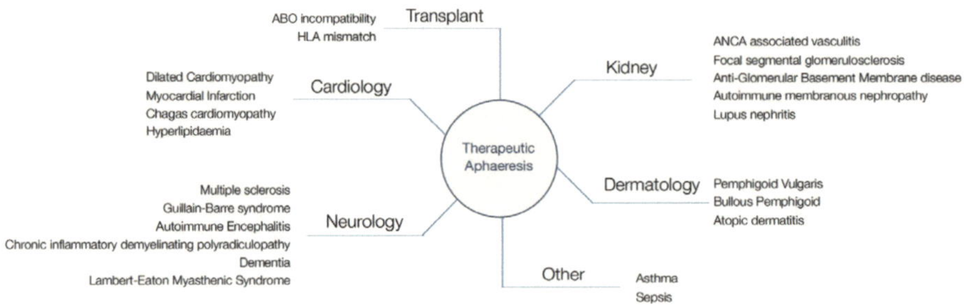

Figure 1. Range of conditions in which therapeutic apheresis has been used.

2. Procedure

Despite the large number of IA columns available the basic principle of the procedure is similar throughout. As with other extracorporeal therapies central venous access is required in order to ensure an adequate blood flow of ~100–150 ml/min through the system. The system itself is a closed system using single use tubing passing the blood from the central venous catheter to a plasma or cell separator, through the column, before combining with the blood components and back into the body via the central venous catheter (**Figure 2**).

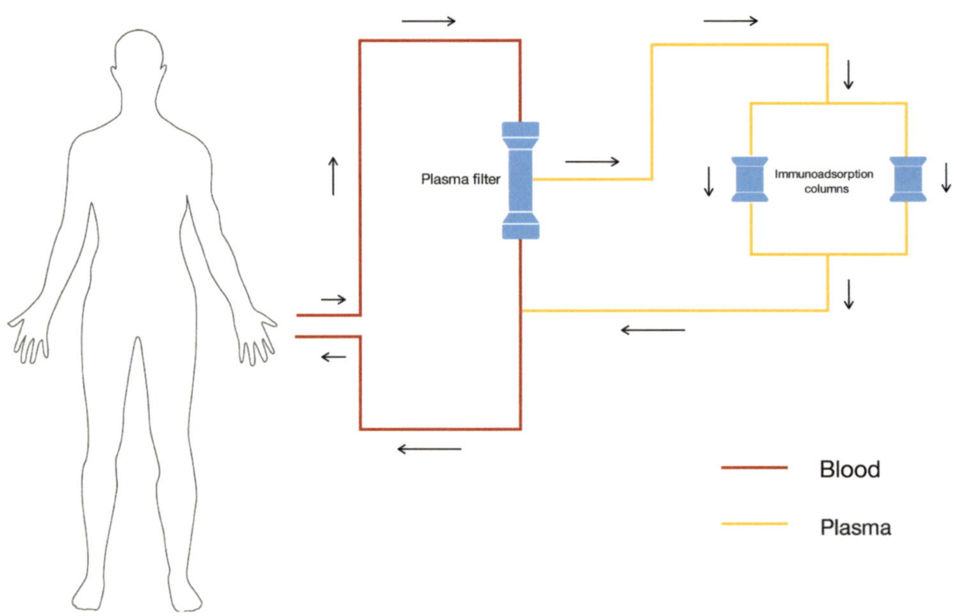

Figure 2. Immunoadsorption schematic. Blood first passes to plasma filter. Plasma then passes on to immunoadsorption column before returning to patient. Schematic shown is dual column system. As the plasma is passing through one column, the second column is being regenerated. Once the first column is saturated the flow switches to the second column whilst the first is then regenerated.

The initial step in immunoadsorption is therefore separation of plasma from the blood cells. Currently there are a number of machines available for this; the *Art* Universal plasma separator (Fresenius Medical Care), Octo *Nova* plasma separator (Diamed Medizintechnik), COBE Spectra Apheresis system (Terumo), Plasmaflo OP plasma separator (Asahi Kasei Medical Co.) and the COMTEC cell separator (Fresenius Medical Care).

The plasma then flows through to a second machine and into the immunoadsorption column. A number of machines are on the market for this stage of the procedure in order to monitor and regulate the plasma flow through the column; the Adsorption-Desorption-Automated system (ADAsorb, Medicap Clinic GmbH) being the most common dual column system in use today.

In dual column systems, the plasma passes through one column whilst the second column is being regenerated. Once the active column has been saturated, the plasma flow switches to the second column whilst the first column itself undergoes regeneration. This system allows for continuous treatment of the plasma with no theoretical upper limit on the number of plasma volumes that can be treated.

All columns share the same fundamental basics, with a matrix containing the molecule used to bind the required immunoglobulin. It is through this matrix that the plasma flows with immunoglobulin binding as it passes. The binding molecule in each adsorber come from a number of different sources both synthetic and organic and this heterogeneity adds to the versatility of the treatment. For example, protein A is found in the cell wall of *Staphylococcus aureus* and has been shown to bind immunoglobulins and in particular IgG with high affinity. It has the ability to bind all the subclasses of IgG with very little binding of other immunoglobulins [1]. The Globaffin adsorber, in contrast, uses a synthetic peptide (Peptid-GAM) to bind IgG with high affinity, and again, all subclasses [2] (**Table 1**).

Treatment prescriptions for immunoadsorption are based on plasma volumes with differing recommendations for each condition as discussed below. Depending on the condition being treated, sessions can be daily or intermittent, again discussed below for each indication. For most patients, plasma volume can be calculated using the Kaplan formula; estimated plasma volume = (0.065 × Weight (kg)) × (1 − Haematocrit) [3]. This formula however does assume a normal body mass index with decreasing accuracy for outliers. In these situations, particularly relevant in patients with nephrotic syndrome and morbid obesity, body composition monitoring may be of benefit to assess a patient's normohydration/ideal body weight (IW). This can then be used in the Kaplan formula for a more accurate plasma volume:

$$\text{Estimated plasma volume} = \left(0.065 \times \text{IW}\,(\text{kg})\right) \times (1 - \text{Haematocrit}). \tag{1}$$

All patients undergoing IA need anticoagulation. This usually takes the form of citrate sodium with IV calcium replacement. In our centre we use 10 ml 10% calcium gluconate for every 2 L of plasma treated. Heparin can also be used as an anticoagulation although generally in combination with sodium citrate and not as the sole agent.

Immunoadsorption type	Binding material	Available columns
Selective	Sepsis and septic shock	Pocard Toxipak
	CRP	PentraSorb CRP
	C1q	Miro
	ABO	Gylcosorb ABO and ABO Adsopak
	PDCM075 and PDCM349	Coraffin
	IgE	IgEnio
	Cholesterol	DALI
	Lipoproteins and macromolecules	MONET
	LDL cholesterol	Pocard LDL Lipopak
	Lipoprotein(a)	Pocard Lp (a) Lipopak
Semi-selective	Staphylococcal protein A	Immunosorba
	Sheep anti-human Ig	Therasorb and Ig-Adsopak
	Peptide-GAM	Globaffin and Ligasorb
Non-selective	Phenylalanine	Immunosorba PH
	Tryptophan	Immunosorba TR-350
	Dextran sulphate	Selesorb
Extracorporeal devices	oXiris	Endotoxins and cytokines
	CytoSorb	Cytokines
	Toraymyxin	Endotoxins

Table 1. Immunoadsorption and extracorporeal columns from non-selective to selective showing the wide range of systems available.

All columns are single patient use only. However, the number of times a column can be used differs from single use, such as the Ligasorb (Fresenius Medical Care) up to 2 years for the Globaffin column (Fresenius Medical Care).

Due to the disposable single use consumables and patient specific columns along with the fact that there is no reliance on blood component replacement, the risk of blood borne disease is minimal. However, there is still a theoretical risk cross-infection and pre-therapy screening for blood borne viruses is advisable.

Of note is the contraindication for the use of concomitant angiotensin-converting enzyme inhibitors (ACEi) with the use of columns using a native peptide such as tryptophan immunoadsorption [4]. This is due to the ACEi induced reduction of bradykinin metabolism following its release during IA. In columns using a synthetic peptide such as the Globaffin, this appears to be less of a concern and the use of ACEi is not contraindicated.

3. Immunoadsorption therapy prescription: example

Patient name	....
Date of birth	....
Hospital number	....
Primary disease for treatment	....
Dates of therapy	....
Frequency	Daily/weekly
Plasma volumes to treat	....
Weight	............kg
Plasma volume (PV)	[Body weight (kg) × 0.065] × [1 − Haematocrit] = ... L
Treatment volume	Plasma volumes to treat × PV = ... L
Flow rate	25 ml/min (1.5 L/h)
Expected time	Treatment volume/1.5 L = ... h and .... min
Anticoagulation	Citrate sodium/heparin
	Calcium infusion as per local guidelines
Name of prescriber	....
Signature of prescriber	....
Date	....

4. Immunoadsorption therapy and its use in sepsis

4.1. Definition

Sepsis is defined as life-threatening organ dysfunction caused by a dysregulated host response to infection. The previously used diagnostic criteria of the presence of two or more features of the Systemic Inflammatory Response Syndrome (SIRS) was replaced in 2016 with new consensus definitions (see Box 1) to provide a more reliable diagnostic criteria, improve consistency across clinical trials and facilitate earlier diagnosis and management [5].

Box 1. Diagnosis of Sepsis and Septic Shock according to the "Third International Consensus Definitions for Sepsis and Septic Shock" [5].

- Sepsis is defined as life-threatening organ dysfunction caused by a dysregulated host response to infection.
- Organ dysfunction can be identified as an acute change in total SOFA score_2 points consequent to the infection.

- The baseline SOFA score can be assumed to be zero in patients not known to have pre-existing organ dysfunction.
- ASOFAscore_2 reflects an overall mortality risk of approximately10%in a general hospital population with suspected infection. Even patients presenting with modest dysfunction can deteriorate further, emphasizing the seriousness of this condition and the need for prompt and appropriate intervention, if not already being instituted.
- In lay terms, sepsis is a life-threatening condition that arises when the body's response to an infection injures its own tissues and organs.
- Patients with suspected infection who are likely to have a prolonged ICU stay or to die in the hospital can be promptly identified at the bedside with qSOFA, ie, alteration in mental status, systolic blood pressure_100 mmHg, or respiratory rate_22/min.
- Septic shock is a subset of sepsis in which underlying circulatory and cellular/metabolic abnormalities are profound enough to substantially increase mortality.
- Patients with septic shock can be identified with a clinical construct of sepsis with persisting hypotension requiring vasopressors to maintain MAP_65 mmHg and having a serum lactate level >2 mmol/L (18 mg/dL) despite adequate volume resuscitation. With these criteria, hospital mortality is in excess of 40%.

4.2. Incidence

As a result of these changing definitions and the inherent clinical heterogeneity of sepsis syndromes, precise incidences are often difficult to estimate. A point prevalence study from the Netherlands in 2004 using the older diagnostic criteria found an incidence of 0.054% of the population, 0.61% of hospital admissions but 11% of ICU admissions [6]. A post hoc analysis of patients in Australian and New Zealand Intensive Care Units found that a significantly larger proportion of patients met the criteria for diagnosis of sepsis when using the new (SOFA) versus the old (SIRS) definitions, 87.1 versus 58.9% [7]. It is apparent that despite these difficulties in classification, the incidence of sepsis is increasing, likely secondary to an ageing population and the increase in risk factors such as cancer, chemotherapy and other chronic diseases.

4.3. Pathophysiology

The pathogenesis of sepsis remains incompletely understood. The progression of a simple localised infection through to septic shock and multiorgan dysfunction involves a complex interplay of proinflammatory and anti-inflammatory cytokines and coagulation factors which result in endothelial disruption, alterations in fluid homeostasis, tissue oedema, reduced end organ perfusion and eventually multiorgan failure. These interactions and their ultimate clinical sequelae depend on factors related to the antecedent infection, the host's response, the presence of comorbidity and the extremes of age, and are mitigated by, and often worsened by, iatrogenic interventions aimed at halting and reversing these conditions. A not infrequent clinical syndrome ensues, familiar to most Intensive Care Physicians, of a patient mechanically ventilated on the intensive care unit, requiring high dose vasopressors and renal replacement therapy. Inoculation with a virulent pathogen triggers a cascade of events resulting in the activation of the innate immune response and the release of proinflammatory cytokines. The initial host response is triggered by recognition of the invading pathogen's molecular signatures (Pathogen Associated Molecular Patterns) or the tissue damage caused by the cellular apoptosis such as ATP and mitochondrial DNA (Damage Associated Molecular Patterns). These activate receptors (Toll-like receptors and C-type lectin receptors) and result in the systemic release of proinflammatory cytokines, predominantly interleukin-1 (Il-1), Il-6 and tumour necrosis factor alpha [8].

This release of cytokines triggers further activation of the hosts immune response, resulting in migration of macrophages and activating further cells of the innate immune systems to release more cytokines, proteases and reactive oxygen species. Coagulation pathways are also activated with widespread activation by tissue factor and by impaired intrinsic anticoagulants such as protein C. It is thought that protease-activated receptors (PAR's) that result from widespread thrombin deposition may play a role in endothelial-cell barrier function breakdown and widespread inflammation [9]. Activation of these pathways results in widespread endothelial release of inducible nitric oxide synthase and this along with other mechanisms causes vasoplegia resulting in systemic hypotension and compensatory activation of the renin angiotensin pathway. These perturbations and the responding compensatory pathways result in a high incidence of acute kidney injury in sepsis with estimates ranging from 19% in 'moderate sepsis' to 51% in 'septic shock' [10].

4.4. Treatment

The mainstay of management for sepsis continues to be early recognition and the institution of appropriate antimicrobial therapy and supportive care. A retrospective cohort study in 2006 demonstrated an increase in mortality associated with a delay in antibiotics beyond 1 h after the recognition of septic shock and an increasing mortality associated with further delay [11]. The institution of the sepsis six 1-h bundle by the Surviving Sepsis Campaign (www.survivingsepsis.org) aimed to enforce the time critical nature of these interventions with delay in administration of antibiotics associated with an increasing mortality (see Box 2). Despite early enthusiasm and uptake for the use of goal directed therapies in critical care, more recent randomised controlled trials have not demonstrated their superiority to standard care in patients admitted to the ICU with sepsis. Supportive management will often involve the use of vasopressor and inotropic support, mechanical ventilation and continuous renal replacement therapy.

Box 2. Surviving Sepsis Campaign Hour-1 bundle of care.

- Measure lactate level
- Obtain blood cultures before administering antibiotics.
- Administer broad-spectrum antibiotics.
- Begin rapid administration of 30 mL/kg crystalloid for hypotension or lactate level ≥ 4 mmol/L.
- Apply vasopressors if hypotensive during or after fluid resuscitation to maintain MAP ≥ 65 mm Hg.

There is ongoing debate as to the role of corticosteroid therapy in sepsis and septic shock. Recent randomised controlled trials have demonstrated that hydrocortisone improves the resolution of septic shock in patients who are refractory to vasopressors but the evidence for improvement in mortality is mixed. In the Activated Protein C and Corticosteroids for Human Septic Shock (APROCCHS) Trial there was evidence of an improvement in 90 day mortality in patients treated with hydrocortisone 200 mg daily with fludrocortisone compared to placebo (43.0 versus 49.1%) [12]. The Adjunctive Corticosteroid Treatment in Critically Ill Patients with Septic Shock (ADRENAL) trial however failed to demonstrate a mortality difference in patients treated with hydrocortisone 200 mg daily versus placebo (27.9 versus 28.8%) [13]. Both trials however showed that the use of hydrocortisone was associated with a faster resolution of septic shock and the use of vasopressors as secondary outcomes. It is possible that the difference in the primary outcome of mortality between these two landmark studies may be the additional use of mineralocorticoid therapy but it may also be related to the differing patient groups and predicted mortality between the two trials, with the APROCCHS trial demonstrating an improvement in 90 day mortality in patients who were more unwell and with a higher overall mortality [14]. There remains large clinical variation in the use of hydrocortisone therapy in septic shock but it is likely that some clinicians will continue their use judiciously in patients with septic shock refractory to vasopressor support. Beyond the use of steroids there has been much interest in the use of immunomodulatory therapies in the treatment of sepsis. Perhaps the most well studied of these is the use of recombinant human activated protein C (rhAPC). Initially encouraging trials showed a mortality benefit of the use of rhAPC in patients with sepsis and multiorgan dysfunction, felt in part due to its anticoagulant effect mitigating the procoagulant and frequent disseminated intravascular coagulation seen in more severe forms of sepsis [15]. It was also favoured for its anti-inflammatory properties. Unfortunately, despite these early positive trials, subsequent randomised controlled trials failed to show a benefit of rhAPC and it was quickly removed from the market by its manufacturer [16]. Despite improvements in supportive care, sepsis remains a heavy burden on intensive care units worldwide and continues to be associated with a high mortality in critically ill patients with an ongoing need for novel, effective treatments.

4.4.1. Extracorporeal therapy

Given the active role of immune system factors in sepsis there has, over the years, an interest in the use of extracorporeal devices for the removal of these perceived pathogenic components. Toraymyxin is an extracorporeal method of removing endotoxins using the polypeptide polymyxin-B immobilised onto polystyrene fibres. Also known as PMX haemoperfusion (PMX-HP), it was developed in the early 1990s in Japan and approved for use in Europe in 2002. Since that time, it has been used in a significant number of patients with sepsis or septic shock in ICU. However, evidence for its benefit has been inconsistent and a recent meta-analysis has concluded that there is no strong evidence for its routine use [17].

Other extracorporeal systems for use in the setting of sepsis include CytoSorb and oXiris. CytoSorb is a single use column designed for the removal of excessive cytokines. Despite showing a significant reduction in circulating cytokine levels, there is a lack of evidence to show an improvement in outcomes and as such its use it not currently recommended by regulatory bodies such as the National Institute for Health and Care Excellence (NICE) in the United Kingdom [18, 19]. oXiris is an acrylonitrile and methalylsulfonate (AN69) membrane that has been shown to remove both endotoxins and cytokines *in vitro* and is now the subject of a number of randomly controlled trials investigating its benefit clinically [20].

4.4.2. Immunoadsorption in sepsis

In a recent study, IA was used to selectively remove LSP, IL-6 and C5a in 11 adult patients (and 22 controls) with severe sepsis admitted to ICU. The treatment was well tolerated and patients had no ongoing anticoagulation abnormalities following IA therapy. All three factors were markedly reduced following treatment in the IA group, in addition to which C-reactive protein (CRP) and fibrinogen were reduced to 27 and 36% of their initial values. There was no change to the inflammatory factors in the control group. Using a number of markers of disease severity, those patients in the treatment group showed a meaningful improvement compared to the control group. Number of days ventilated and the number of days in ICU were both significantly less in the treatment group as was the amount of norepinephrine needed. There was a tendency to a reduction in the number needing renal replacement therapy although this was not statistically significant. Acute Physiology and Chronic Health Evaluation II (APACHE II), mean Sequential Organ Failure Assessment (SOFA) and mean Multiple Organ Failure (MOF) scores all improved significantly more in the treatment group compared to the control group [21].

This pilot study shows that IA appears to be safe and tolerated well in patients with severe sepsis with significant objective improvements as measure both biochemically and clinically.

5. Other indications for the use of immunoadsorption

5.1. Nephrology

5.1.1. Transplantation

As patients reach end-stage renal disease (ESRD) and require renal replacement therapy (RRT), dialysis can be a lifeline but long-term outcomes remain poor. Renal transplantation can not only improve a patients' quality of life but also extend it beyond that of dialysis [22–24]. Traditionally renal transplantation matching has been based on a close Human Leukocyte Antigen (HLA) match and ABO compatibility. With an ever-increasing population reaching ESRD and necessitating RRT but with the continued donor kidney shortage, methods to allow for a relaxation of these matching criteria can greatly increase the uptake of renal transplantation [25].

5.1.1.1. ABO-incompatibility

Early attempts to use transplantation in the presence of ABO-incompatibility (ABOi) proved unsuccessful and its use was contraindicated for many years due to the risk of hyperacute and acute allograft rejection [26–30]. The ABO blood group system was first described by Landsteiner in 1901 [31]. Patients can have A, B, both or neither antigens on their erythrocytes along with antibodies to the antigens they do not possess. For example, patients with blood group A will have A antigens on their erythrocytes, and antibodies to B antigen (anti-B) in their plasma. Since the 1980s there has been an increased understanding of the underlying mechanisms of ABOi rejection. This rejection is triggered by the recognition by the recipient antibodies (anti-A or anti-B) of the corresponding A and/or B blood group antigen on the graft endothelium. Earlier attempts at removing these antibodies to allow for ABOi transplantation involved intensive perioperative plasma exchange, splenectomy and judicious immunosuppression with resulting high mortality and morbidity but with little improvement in outcomes [26].

Given the anti-A/B blood group antigens are of the IgG and IgM subclass, the use of immunoadsorption offers the ability to selectively remove these antibodies and there is now strong evidence for it use with long-term follow up [26, 32].

In 2001, Tydén et al. published a protocol utilising immunoadsorption and rituximab as an adjunct to standard triple therapy immunosuppression to significantly reduce the blood group antigens prior to transplantation. This regimen has now been used extensively, particularly in Europe, with excellent long-term outcomes, comparable to ABO compatible transplantation [33–38].

5.1.1.2. HLA mismatch

In a similar manner to ABOi, recipient antibodies directed against donor HLA are a major cause of graft rejection [39, 40]. Unfortunately, a large number of patients on the transplant waiting list will have these antibodies as a result of blood transfusions, pregnancy or previous transplants [41–44]. As with ABOi, the presence of these antibodies can reduce the chance of a patient receiving a transplant and increase time on the waiting list. Methods have therefore been sought to desensitise patients in order to improve their chances of a suitable match and to improve outcomes post transplantation. Most strategies at present employ plasma exchange and IVIg with good results showing that the removal of these antibodies can confer a favourable outcome for the patient [45]. Given its more selective nature, IA offers an alternative to plasma exchange and has been used in a number of small studies with varying degrees of success.

In 1996, Higgins et al. used IA in 13 highly sensitised patients prior to transplantation. Three patients' grafts failed due to rejection and six of the remaining 10 patients had reversible episodes of rejection [46]. Since that time there have been a number of studies showing IA is a viable therapy for desensitisation prior to transplantation [47, 48].

5.1.2. Autoimmune membranous nephropathy

Despite being a rare disease, autoimmune membranous nephropathy (MN) is among the most common causes of adult nephrotic syndrome worldwide [49–54]. In the majority of patients, it is associated with the M-Type Phospholipase 2 Receptor autoantibody (Anti-PLA_2R), discovered in 2009 [55]. Since that time there has been a tremendous increase in our understanding of the disease process although this has yet to translate into disease specific therapies for patient. At present, the current standard of care involves the use of a rotating regimen involving high dose steroids and cyclophosphamide over a 6 month period, known as the Ponticelli regimen, and has been in use in various forms for almost 20 years [56–58]. This regimen was developed before the discovery of the anti-PLA_2R but with the belief that the condition was an autoimmune disease. It takes a blunderbuss approach to suppressing the immune system with good clinical response but with a significant side-effect burden both in the short term and the long term.

The anti-PLA_2R antibody itself is an IgG antibody and current evidence appears to suggest that it is a pathogenic antibody [55, 59–62]. This makes it not only a good biomarker for disease activity and response to treatment but potentially a target of treatment in itself.

Before the discovery of anti-PLA_2R, Esnault et al. use protein A immunoadsorption on four patients with membranous nephropathy. All four patients had an improvement in their proteinuria with very little side-effects. However, the study only had a short follow up period of 4 weeks and no antibody data [63].

A clinical trial using the Fresenius Peptide GAM immunoadsorption column Globaffin has at the time of writing completed recruitment and treatment of 12 patients. The Globaffin column has a specificity for IgG antibodies of all subclasses and as such is expected to render the patients anti-PLA_2R negative. Follow up is ongoing but unpublished reports suggest that this is a promising new therapy for autoimmune membranous nephropathy with a drastically reduced side-effect burden when compared to the Ponticelli regimen [64].

5.1.3. *Anti-glomerular basement membrane disease*

Anti-glomerular basement membrane disease (anti-GBM), also known as Goodpasture's syndrome, is a rare life-threatening autoimmune disease, typically presenting as rapidly progressive crescentic glomerulonephritis and lung haemorrhage. It is invariably fatal unless treated promptly with an intensive regime of immunomodulation with high dose steroids, immunosuppression and plasma exchange. With current treatment standards mortality has improved although renal impairment remains a significant challenge [58, 65]. Patients who are dialysis dependent on presentation unfortunately rarely recover renal function [58, 66, 67].

The disease is associated with the pathogenic anti-GBM autoantibodies which are directed against the glomerular basement membrane [68] and in particular the non-collagenous domain 1 (NC1) of α3 chain of type IV collagen. These antibodies are predominantly IgG, occasionally IgM, and can be readily detected in the circulation as well as being demonstrated along the glomerular basement membrane on histology, a combined finding that is confirmation of the diagnosis [65].

Treatment strategies are aimed at the removal of the pathogenic antibody with oral prednisolone at the earliest clinical suspicion of the disease. Once a diagnosis has been confirmed, cyclophosphamide is started as is plasma exchange. Plasma exchange continues for 14 sessions or until the serum antibody is negative. If a patient goes into remission, unlike many other autoimmune diseases, patients rarely have a return of the antibody or relapse of the condition [58].

Given its superiority in removing antibodies compared to plasma exchange, immunoadsorption provides a promising alternative to the rapid reduction of the offending autoantibodies. Currently there are no RCTs investigating the efficacy of IA versus standard of care and for many years evidence was conflicting based on small case series from around the world using different adsorbers.

The first published treatment of Goodpastures using IA was in 1985 by Bygren et al. using protein A immunoadsorption resulting in a dramatic clinical improvement in a patient who had failed to respond to plasma exchange [69]. In four Chinese patients using protein A IA, all saw a reduction in their antibody levels and resolution of their pulmonary haemorrhage. One patient managed to recover renal function in order to stop haemodialysis but the three others remained dialysis dependent. All three of these had 100% crescent formation on biopsy [70]. However, two patients with dialysis dependent anti-GBM disease treated with protein A immunoadsorption by Esnault et al. showed no clinical improvement at all [71].

Two patients treated in Spain showed a reduction in the circulating antibody and improvement in respiratory symptoms but no renal improvement [72]. A Swedish study treating three patients with Goodpasture's also showed no clinical improvement using IA (Excorim, Sweden) although all patients were dialysis dependent on initiation of the treatment [73]. Two patients from Vienna were successfully treated using the TheraSorb adsorber, one of whom regained renal function despite presenting with 100% crescents on histology [74].

The largest series to date though, reveals some encouraging results. Biesenbach et al. treated 10 consecutive patients using either the TheraSorb (Miltenyi Biotec, Germany) or the Immunosorba (Fresenius Medical Care, Germany), treating 2.5–3.0 PV per session. All patients had adjunctive prednisolone and cyclophosphamide. All 10 patients were rendered anti-GBM antibody negative within nine sessions and with greater efficiency than demonstrated in PE. Two patients were initially treated with plasma exchange but switched to IA when the antibody failed to reduce. Clinical improvement was seen in both pulmonary haemorrhage and in renal impairment, with three of six patients who had initially presented with dialysis dependency managing to recover renal function. One patient died of fungal infection after the antibody had become negative but otherwise the safety profile was acceptable with no major adverse events recorded [75].

5.1.4. Lupus nephritis

Systemic lupus erythematous (SLE) is an autoimmune disease affecting multiple organs with up to 60% of patients having renal involvement (Lupus Nephritis) [76]. SLE is caused by a loss of immune tolerance leading to the production of autoantibodies, such as anti-double-stranded DNA (anti-dsDNA) autoantibodies, and the development of immune complexes [77–79].

The current standard of care is the use of intravenous cyclophosphamide therapy and is aimed at the inhibition of formation, and reduction of, these pathogenic antibodies [58].

There are now multiple case series, showing a favourable response to IA with a reduction in proteinuria and anti-dsDNA levels, and disease activity as characterised by the Systemic Lupus Activity Measure (SLAM) and the Systemic Lupus Erythematosus Disease Activity Index (SLEDAI) [80–89]. Many of these studies have treated patients with severe disease activity resistant to immunosuppression with very few side effects. As yet there are no RCTs investigating the use of IA versus immunosuppression alone or in combination. Despite this, the use of IA has shown promise as an alternative or adjunctive treatment in lupus nephritis in both the short and long term.

5.1.5. Focal segmental glomerulosclerosis

Focal segmental glomerulosclerosis (FSGS) is a histological diagnosis of a heterogeneous group of conditions. It is the most common cause of adult nephrotic syndrome in the US and one of the most common causes worldwide and its incidence is rising [54, 90]. It is separated into either primary or idiopathic FSGS or secondary FSGS. Secondary FSGS can be further subdivided into genetic, virus-associated, drug-induced or adaptive FSGS [91].

Given this heterogeneity, a sound pathogenic basis of the disease has been elusive. The initiation of the disease process undoubtedly follows a number of different routes, all with resultant podocyte injury. In primary FSGS an immunologic cause has long been suspected with a number of circulating factors now identified as potential candidates such as the IgG anti-CD40 autoantibody although further work is needed in this area [92].

Based on this supposition, the use of immunoadsorption both for primary disease and for recurrent disease post-transplant has been used with varying degrees of success [93, 94].

Haas et al. used IA in five patients with native kidney disease and three patients with recurrent disease in their grafts. Six patients used protein-A IA (Immuno-adsorba, Excorim, Sweden) and two patients with an anti-IgG column (Ig-TheraSorb, Germany). Patients initially had five sessions within 10 days at 2.5 plasma volumes per session. If proteinuria did not improve by more than 50% in this time they underwent another cycle. In four of the eight patients, proteinuria reduced by more than 50% although the mean time to relapse was only 21 days. Following relapse, patients had a further cycle of IA which did appear to provide a benefit with one patient having stable remission for 1.5 years and a second patient being stable for 2 years. However, of the two others who had initially responded, one became resistant to treatment and the other lost his graft after 3 months [93].

LDL-apheresis has also shown some promise with reports from Japan suggesting it may have a role in not only reducing cholesterol, triglycerides and low-density lipoprotein but also proteinuria and an improvement in renal function [95–97]. This has led the ASFA to classify FSGS as a category III condition with grade 2C evidence (Optimum role of apheresis therapy is not yet established based on weak evidence and decision making should be individualized) [98].

5.1.6. ANCA associated vasculitis

Antineutrophil cytoplasmic autoantibody (ANCA)-associated vasculitis (AAV) is an autoimmune disorder affecting small vessels. It can involve any organ although has a predilection for the upper airways, lungs and kidneys. It is a chronic relapsing-remitting disease following the general pattern of many autoimmune diseases with a genetic component, environmental or infective trigger and the formation of autoantibodies resulting in an immune cascade and subsequent injury [99, 100].

Prior to the introduction of steroids and immunosuppression, the disease was invariably fatal [101]. Nowadays the vast majority of patients will survive but given the judicious amounts of steroids and immunosuppression required for remission, many patients will have iatrogenic complications of the treatment itself [102–106].

The disease is associated with the formation of autoantibodies to either myeloperoxidase (MPO) or proteinase 3 (PR3) found on the granules of neutrophils and the lysosomes of monocytes in 90% of patients. As well as being a biomarker for the disease, there is evidence to suggest that it has at least some pathogenic features, particularly in animal models of the disease [99]. Along with this and the fact that it is an IgG antibody [107], a number of groups have investigated the use of immunoadsorption in the treatment of AAV. There does appear to be effective removal of the antibodies, however numbers in these studies are limited, there is concomitant use of immunosuppression and the results inconsistent [71, 73, 108, 109].

5.2. Cardiology

5.2.1. Hyperlipidaemia

Familial hypercholesterolaemia (FH) is an autosomal dominant genetic defect resulting in raised serum cholesterol and an increased risk of cardiovascular disease. Patients can present as either homozygous or heterozygous FH, with homozygous patients exhibiting a more severe phenotype. If left untreated patients with FH have a significantly increased risk of cardiovascular disease. The majority of patients exhibit a mutation in the LDL receptor, although mutations in the Apo B and proprotein convertase subtilisin/kexin type 9 genes have also been detected [110–112].

Initially patients should be treated with lifestyle changes and aggressive statin therapy, however, in many patients this will not suffice. In the United Kingdom, the National Institute for Health and Care Excellence (NICE) suggests considering the use of IA for adults and young patients with homozygous familial hypercholesterolaemia (FH) and in heterozygous FH progressive, symptomatic coronary heart disease despite maximal medical therapy. This is generally on a weekly or biweekly regimen and given the frequency, an arterio-vascular fistula is recommended [113].

In the United States (US), LDL-apheresis is approved for use by the Food and Drug Administration (FDA) in patients who have not responded to treatment after 6 months. In homozygous FH non-response is defined patients with an LDL cholesterol of above 300 mg/dL or a non-HDL-cholesterol level of above 330 mg/dL. In heterozygous FH, non-response is defined as HDL-cholesterol above 300 mg/dL and 0-1 risk factors. In patients with established coronary heart disease, cardiovascular disease or diabetes, an HDL-cholesterol level of above 160 mg/dL is used [114].

Lipoprotein(a) is a plasma protein consisting of a low-density lipoprotein (LDL) covalently bonded to an apolipoprotein(a) molecule. Elevated lipoprotein(a) levels have consistently been reported as an association for increased risk of cardiovascular disease although much of this has been a causal link. However, given the weight of evidence for its involvement in cardiovascular disease, the European Atherosclerosis Society Consensus Panel on the treatment of lipoprotein(a) recommends treatment to ensure the serum level is below 50 mg/dL [115]. Therapeutic agents are limited with the standard therapy being niacin, alone or in combination with statins, with little impact from lifestyle changes. In patients unresponsive to or intolerant of pharmacological solutions immunoadsorption provides an alternative therapy. European Atherosclerosis Society Consensus Panel also suggests considering IA therapy in young or middle-aged patients with progressive coronary disease and significantly raised plasma lipoprotein(a) levels [115]. In the US, apheresis is approved for use by the FDA in heterozygous FH patients unresponsive to medical therapy after 6 months with an LDL-cholesterol level of above 200 mg/dL and lipoprotein(a) above 50 mg/dL [114].

Homozygous FH is a category I condition whilst heterozygous FH is a category II condition with both having a grade 1A recommendation as per the American Society for Apheresis (ASFA) guidelines on the use of therapeutic apheresis in clinical practice. Lipoprotein(a) hyperproteinaemia is a category II condition with a 1B grade recommendation. A category I condition is a disorder in which apheresis is the accepted first line therapy and a category II condition is one in which apheresis is the accepted second line therapy, as a stand-alone modality or as an adjunct to other treatment. A grade 1A recommendation is defined as a strong recommendation based on high quality evidence and applicable to most patients without reservation. A grade 1B recommendation is a strong recommendation based on moderate quality evidence and can be applied to the majority of patients in most circumstances [98].

5.2.2. Dilated cardiomyopathy

Dilated cardiomyopathy (DCM) is a progressive disease that is a major cause of heart failure worldwide with a high mortality and morbidity. Despite treatment it remains one of the main precipitants to heart transplants in adults [116, 117]. In most patients the cause is unknown, but for a significant proportion it is an autoimmune disease. After years of speculation that there was an autoimmune component to condition, a number of autoantibodies have now been discovered. Evidence now suggests that these autoantibodies, particularly β1-adrenoreceptor autoantibodies (β1-AAB), are pathogenic in nature [118, 119]. Given they are generally of the IgG class, removal of the antibody is particularly amenable to IA and it has now been used successfully in DCM for over 2 decades with a significant body of evidence supporting its use. The first reported case series from 1996 used the Ig-TheraSorb (Baxter, Germany) column to treat eight patients with severe DCM and NYHA class II-IV [120].

Since that time a number of studies have reported on the benefits of IA in DCM both short and long term, with a reduction in circulating antibodies and with clinical improvement [121–128].

Dörffel et al. treated nine patients with NYHA class III or IV and ejection fraction <25%, on 5 consecutive days with the Ig-TheraSorb (Baxter). Here there was a marked reduction in circulating antibody level and an improvement in the patients' dyspnoea. There was no improvement in LVEF in this study although this is likely due to the very short follow up [129]. A longer prospective case control study with a 1-year follow-up expanded on this earlier work. Here 34 patients with an NYHA class II or above significant LV dysfunction and considered candidates for heart transplantation were enrolled. 17 patients received standard medical treatment whilst 17 received adjunctive IA for 5 consecutive days. β1-AAB levels had a highly significant mean reduction of 93.2% at month three with no significant increase within the 1 year follow up. Antibody levels remained unchanged in the control group [123].

At 1 year follow up there was also a marked improvement in the cardiac performance of patients in the control group with a significant increase in their LVEF and a reduction in the left ventricular internal diameter in diastole (LVIDd). At 5 years post-IA there was also a statistically significant improvement in survival for those patients in the treatment group compared to the control group [123].

Long-term data also suggests that the antibodies are slow to reappear. In a study of 108 patients, only 16 (14.6%) had detectable antibodies 3 years post-IA and a further nine (8.3%) had detectable antibodies after 3 years post-IA. In the majority of these patients (76%), the reappearance of the antibody correlated with a deterioration in their clinical symptoms. With this continued antibody remission there continues to be long-term clinical improvement. Some studies show a mortality rate similar to post-transplantation, although with a lower LVEF [119, 121, 128].

Many of these studies have utilised replacement intravenous immunoglobulins at the end of the IA treatment. There has been some suggestion that much of the benefits seen are due to this although there does appear to be clinical and biochemical improvement without IVIg replacement [130].

IA use in dilated cardiomyopathy has a level II category and 1B grade recommendation as per the American Society for Apheresis (ASFA) guidelines on the use of therapeutic apheresis in clinical practice. A level II category is defined as a disorder in which apheresis is the accepted second line therapy or first line in conjunction with other treatments. A grade 1B recommendation is defined as a strong recommendation with moderate quality of evidence and can be applied to the majority of patients without reservation [98].

5.2.3. Myocardial infarction

Despite ever increasing survival following acute MI, post-MI morbidity continues to present patients with a modest prognosis. Interest in the inflammatory response following an MI has gained traction in recent years and in particular the role C-reactive protein (CRP) plays in ongoing myocardial damage. Along with this, elevated CRP is a poor risk factor for all-cause mortality, major adverse cardiac events and recurrent MIs [131, 132]. Experimental animal models have shown that inhibition of CRP following induced MI results in a smaller infarct area although this therapeutic molecule is still in early development and not yet humanised [133, 134]. Immunoadsorption now offers the ability to remove CRP with specific adsorbers in early animal models suggesting a benefit. In a study of 10 pigs (five receiving IA and five controls) with induced MI, those pigs who underwent IA had a reduction in the post-MI infarct size and preservation of their cardiac output as measured by LVEF [135]. Given these promising results a clinical trial is now underway in Germany to investigate the benefit of using CRP-specific immunoadsorption in acute ST-elevation MI (STEMI). Unpublished interim analysis suggests that the therapy is safe and well tolerated post-STEMI with promising results on infarct size in relation to CRP reduction. The results of this study have the potential to change management following an MI and subsequent PCI with an improvement in patient morbidity and mortality long-term.

5.2.4. *Chagas cardiomyopathy*

Chagas disease, caused by *Trypanosoma cruzi* (*T. cruzi*), affects ~10 million people per year, predominantly in South America where it is endemic. Of those affected, many have no long-term sequelae but up to 40% can develop Chagas Cardiomyopathy with arrhythmias, heart failure and an increased mortality [136, 137]. The vast majority of patients with Chagas cardiomyopathy are known to possess IgG autoantibodies suggesting an autoimmune component to the disease with the potential to respond to IA therapy. A clinical trial is currently underway to investigate this.

5.3. Neurology

5.3.1. *Multiple sclerosis*

Multiple sclerosis (MS) is the most common chronic inflammatory condition of the central nervous system (CNS) worldwide. It is characterised by demyelination of differing parts of the CNS (space) with different lesions appearing over time. A majority of patients present with visual loss due to optic neuritis although depending on where the lesion is can also present with symptoms such as limb weakness, sensory loss, ataxia or cognitive impairment [138–140]. It is estimated to affect 50–300 per 100,000 with ~2 million people diagnosed worldwide. It is generally a disease of early adulthood and given the impact on mobility and quality of life the disease confers, it represents a significant healthcare burden [141]. There are currently four recognised phenotypes of the condition. Many patients present with a single episode that resolves over time known as a clinically isolated syndrome. Patients who then go on to have further episodes (relapses) are described as having remitting-relapsing MS. Approximately 15% of patients will present with a progressive disease course from onset known as primary progressive MS. The fourth category is the development over time of secondary progressive MS in a proportion of patients with relapsing-remitting MS. The pathogenesis of MS is still not clearly defined although genetic, lifestyle and autoimmune factors are all understood to play a role in the disease [139, 140, 142].

There are now a large number of approved disease modifying medications for the treatment of MS with apheresis reserved for non-responders. In many national guidelines for the treatment of MS, TPE is considered a second line therapy for steroid resistant relapsing-remitting MS [143]. The American Society for Apheresis (ASFA) gives TPE for MS a category II (Disorders for which apheresis is accepted as second-line therapy, either as a standalone treatment or in conjunction with other modes of treatment) based on grade 1B evidence (Strong recommendation, moderate quality evidence) [98]. As early as 1989, IA has been shown to be as effective as TPE in the treatment of MS with an ever-growing body of evidence to support its role [144–149]. However, given the lack of RCTs there has been limited uptake of the therapy. This has led relapsing-remitting MS to be an indication for IA by the ASFA although the lack of RCTs has resulted in it being designated a category III disease with Grade 2C evidence (optimum role of apheresis therapy is not established. Decision making should be individualized. Weak recommendation with low-quality or very low-quality evidence) [98].

5.3.2. Guillain-Barré syndrome

Guillain-Barré syndrome (GBS) is one of the most common causes of acute polyneuropathy worldwide with an incidence of ~1 per 100,000. It is considered an autoimmune disease generally found in association with a preceding infection, initiating an immune cascade that results in an inflammatory demyelinating polyneuropathy or acute motor axonal neuropathy [150]. TPE has been used for a number of years with robust evidence. The ASFA have designated GBS a category I condition with grade 1A evidence (disorders for which apheresis is accepted as first-line therapy, either as a primary standalone treatment or in conjunction with other modes of treatment. Strong recommendation, high-quality evidence) [98]. This has inevitably led researchers to consider IA in GBS.

Evidence for IA suggests that it is a treatment that should be considered as a viable alternative to TPE. Most published studies comparing IA to the standard of therapy, be it TPE, double filtration plasma exchange or IVIG has shown that not only is safety comparable or better, but also efficacy is as comparable. This has led a number of researchers to suggest, given its safety record, that it should be considered instead of TPE as a first line treatment [151–154].

5.3.3. Autoimmune encephalitis

Autoimmune encephalitis is an acute neurological inflammatory condition now known to be caused by a variety of antibodies. Treatment therefore generally takes the form of immunomodulation using steroids, IVIG and TPE. As yet there are no randomly controlled trials investigating the efficacy of IA in autoimmune encephalitis and only retrospective trials.

Dogan Onugoren et al. treated 14 patients with autoimmune encephalitis caused by leucine-rich glioma inactivated 1 (LGI1), contactin-associated protein-2 (CASPR2), *N*-methyl-D-aspartate receptor (NMDAR) and intracellular glutamic acid decarboxylase (GAD) antibodies using either tryptophan and protein A adsorbers. Directly after follow up, nine patients (64%) had improved their Modified Rankin Scale (mRS) score by one or more point and five (35%)

became seizure free. At late follow up, several months after IA therapy, 12 (86%) patients had improved mRS scores [155].

Köhler et al. treated 13 patients with antibodies to NMDAR, GAD, Lgl1 and γ-amino-butyric-acid (GABA) using tryptophan IA. Eleven patients (85%) were noted to have a clinical improvement following IA with a good side effect profile [156].

In a prospective observational case control study treating 10 patients with tryptophan IA and 11 with TPE. 60% of patients in the IA group compared to 67% in the TPE showed a clinical improvement with a reduction of their mRS score of one or more points. There were more adverse events in the TPE group (three in the TPE group and zero in the IA group) [157].

A recent review analysed the published studies comparing IA (25 patients in total) to TPE therapy (57 patients), used alone or in combination with steroids. Here they found that 88% of patients improved following IA treatment with 77% of patients improving with TPE treatment. The effect seemed to be more pronounced for antibodies against the neuronal cell surface compared to intracellular antigens. It was also found to be the safer option with fewer side-effects [158].

Despite the lack of RCTs, the evidence for IA in autoimmune encephalitis is encouraging and would suggest that it should be considered as a therapy.

5.3.4. *Chronic inflammatory demyelinating polyradiculoneuropathy*

Chronic inflammatory demyelinating polyradiculoneuropathy (CIDP) is among the most common chronic neuropathies worldwide. Although the exact pathogenesis remains unknown, it is considered an autoimmune disorder directed against, and causing demyelination of, the myelin sheath. This results in progressive or relapsing distal and peripheral weakness. The condition has a multitude of phenotypes, and with this heterogeneity many consider it a spectrum of disease, as opposed to a single disease [159]. Current treatment aims at immunomodulation with IVIG and steroids the first line therapy with consideration of TPE in non-responders. ASFA guidelines consider CIDP as a category I disorder for treatment with TPE (disorders for which apheresis is accepted as first-line therapy, either as a primary standalone treatment or in conjunction with other modes of treatment) with grade 1B evidence (strong recommendation, moderate quality evidence) [98]. Given the efficacy of TPE, a number of studies have investigated the use of IA in CIDP.

Galldiks et al. treated 10 patients with CIDP unresponsive to standard therapy using a tryptophan-linked polyvinyl alcohol adsorber. Response as measured by the inflammatory neuropathy cause and treatment disability (INCAT) score and improvements in strength, sensation and performance of activities of daily living. Improvements in the INCAT was seen in all but one of the patients. Four of the patients received long-term IA in an outpatient setting with clinical improvement. In three of these four patients, they had previously been treated with TPE and noted no clinical decline on switching to IA [160].

Zinman et al. conducted a randomised, single-blinded study investigating the efficacy of protein A immunoadsorption versus IVIG. Here they treated nine patients with high dose IVIG, four with low IVIG and five with IA. One patient in the high dose IVIG withdrew consent prior to treatment and two patients in the low dose IVIG group died of illness not thought to be related to treatment. Six-month data was not available for one patient in the IA group and two in the IVIG arm. Two months following treatment, four patients (80%) in the IA group were considered responders compared to four out of eight (50%) in the IVIG arm. At 6 months, all four of the patients in the IA group were considered responders compared with three out of six in the IVIG group (100 versus 50%) [161].

More recently a prospective randomly controlled study investigating the efficacy and safety of IA versus TPE, again using the tryptophan-linked polyvinylalcohol adsorber. There were nine patients in each group with no significant differences in baseline characteristics. Clinical improvement was assessed using the INCAT score and the Medical Research Council (MRC) sum score. It was found that four patients (44.4%) in the TPE group responded to treatment compared to six patients (66.7%) in the IA group. In the IA group, 100% of the patients had an improvement in their MRC sum scores and four patients out of six patients (66.7%) [162].

Despite these small numbers, IA has shown promising results especially when considering the majority of the patients included in the studies were patients who had already failed standard therapy. The safety profile was comparable to TPE and IVIG and albeit with limited study populations, appeared to be as, if not more, efficacious than the current standard therapy.

5.3.5. Dementia

Dementia represents an increasing problem for healthcare systems worldwide, exacerbated by an aging problem. The most common form, Alzheimer's disease, is characterised by the deposition of β-amyloid plaques and neurofibrillary tangles. The exact cause of the disease remains unknown and given the heterogenous nature of the condition it is likely to be multifactorial. There can also be some overlap in patients with both Alzheimer's disease and Vascular dementia, a disease resulting from damage to the vasculature of the brain. Research has suggested there can be an autoimmune component to some dementia patients with the discovery of autoantibodies against the β_1-adrenergic receptor (β_1-AR) and the β_2-adrenergic receptor (β_2-AR) present in up to 59% of dementia patients [163, 164].

Hempel et al. treated eight patients with immunoadsorption; all patients were anti-β_1-AR positive and five were also anti-β_2-AR positive. Patients treated for 4 consecutive days saw a reduction in anti-β_1-AR levels of 96% compared to only 78% in those treated for 2–3 consecutive days. Those patients treated with 4 days of IA also saw a sustained elimination of antibody over the course of the study but in those treated for a shorter time period saw a rebound of the antibody level. Cognitive function was assessed using a range of tests including the Mini-Mental State Examination (MMSE), Alzheimer's Disease Assessment scale (ADAS; cognitive and non-cognitive), Bayer Activities of Daily Living (Bayer-ADL), Clinical Global Impression Scale (CGI), Geriatric Depression Scale (GDS) and the Short Cognitive Performance Test (SKT). They found that over the course of the study, those treated for 4 days had stabilisation of their cognitive function. Those treated for only 2–3 days suffered from declining cognition [165].

This is a limited study with a small number of patients but its promise has led to a number of current ongoing studies to investigate further.

5.3.6. Lambert-Eaton myasthenic syndrome

Lambert-Eaton myasthenic syndrome (LEMS) is a rare autoimmune disease resulting in muscle weakness, autonomic dysfunction and areflexia. Up to 60% of patients with LEMS will also be found to have a carcinoma, with small cell lung cancer (SCLC) making up the vast majority of these patients. Pathogenic antibodies to voltage-gated calcium channels (VGCC) have been found in 80–90% of patients and up to 100% in patients with SCLC. Current therapy consists of 3,4-diaminopyridine as first line and treatment of any underlying malignancy. Second line treatment involves the addition of pyridostigmine to the 3,4-diaminopyridine or converting to azathioprine and prednisolone. In the case of severe weakness TPE or IVIG can also be considered [166]. There are also a number of very small case series describing the use of IA in refractory LEMS.

Sauter et al. describe the case of a young man with rapidly progressive weakness, muscular atrophy and cerebellar dysfunction initially treated with thymectomy for presumed malignancy and pulsed prednisolone with some resolution of symptoms and a reduction in anti-VGCC antibodies titres. Further treatment with Azathioprine and IVIG was initiated with some improvement clinically although this was not sustained and corresponded with a rise in his antibody titre. IA was performed on 3 consecutive days every 6 weeks with a decrease in antibody level over this time and an improvement symptomatically, especially in regards to gait [167]. Baggi et al. treated three patients unresponsive to immunosuppression and plasma exchange with IA. All patient showed clinical improvement with one patient regaining the ability to walk and one reaching pharmacological remission [168]. Batchelor et al. treated 13 paraneoplastic patients one of whom had LEMS characterised as bilateral ptosis and proximal limb weakness. They received a total of six IA sessions (two per week for 3 weeks) with a protein A adsorber. In the patient with LEMS, clinical improvement was seen with resolution of the ptosis and the recovery of muscle strength allowing her to climb stairs and walk unaided again. There was also a significant reduction in the anti-VGCC antibody titre from 458 to 25 pmol/L [169]. Ishikawa et al. treated a 75 year-old man with gait disturbance and somnolence diagnosed as LEMS. Anti-VGCC titre was initially over 11,000 pmol/L but the use of a phenylalanine adsorber column along with concomitant prednisolone resulted in a significant reduction in his antibody titre and subsequent clinical improvement [170].

There are currently no RCT or prospective trial data for the use of IA in LEMS. However, in patients who are non-responsive to standard therapy or in whom immunosuppression or TPE are contraindicated, there is limited data to suggest that IA can be considered an alternative.

5.4. Dermatology

5.4.1. Pemphigoid vulgaris

Pemphigoid vulgaris (PV) is a potentially fatal autoimmune blistering condition of the skin and mucous membranes. It is associated with pathogenic IgG autoantibodies to the desmosomal cadherins; desmoglein 1 (Dsg1) and desmoglein 3 (Dsg3) [171–173]. Treatment and management of PV can be challenging. Currently treatment consists of oral steroids alone or in combination with dapsone and immunosuppression such as azathioprine, methotrexate or cyclophosphamide. This has dramatically improved survival but there is significant morbidity as a result of the side-effects from these therapies [174].

A number of groups have now used IA with differing adsorbers and protocols. A tryptophan-linked polyvinylalcohol adsorber was used to treat seven patients with severe PV. There was a significant reduction in circulating antibodies and clinical improvement seen in the pemphigoid lesions and a reduction in steroid and immunosuppression required [175]. Protein A immunoadsorption has also been used with the first study describing its use in 2003. Here four patients were treated using IA as an additional treatment to steroids. All patients saw an improvement in their pemphigoid lesions and significant reduction in their antibody titres [176]. Further, nine patients were treated with a modified protocol by Shimanovich et al. with a higher dose of adjunctive steroids and either azathioprine or mycophenolate mofetil. All patients showed a significant reduction in antibody levels and clinically, with remission reported up to 26 months after treatment [177]. Protein A immunoadsorption has also been used in combination with Rituximab and IVIg with positive results [178] and in patients with longstanding disease resistant to multiple therapies [179]. In the largest trial for IA in PV, IA was used in combination with Rituximab in 23 patients. Seventeen patients using protein A IA (Immunosorba) and six patients using polyclonal anti-human IgG sheep antibodies coupled to sepharose (Thera-Sorb). IA was given more frequently than previous protocols with 1000 mg Rituximab given on days 4 and 24. This resulted in a significant reduction in antibody tires in all patients. At 6 months, 16 (70%) of the patients were in complete remission and five (22%) were in partial remission. A relatively low relapse rate of six patients was seen over the follow up period requiring either retreatment with IA, Rituximab or immunosuppression [180].

Given the antibodies to Dsg1 and Dsg3 are IgG, Eming et al. used the Globaffin (Fresenius, Germany), an IgG specific column to treat PV in four patients. All patients experienced a reduction in antibody levels of up to 70% and a marked improvement clinically [181]. Behzad et al. used the Globaffin column in combination with Rituximab in 10 difficult to control PV patients in a retrospective study. Six months after treatment, 8 out of the 10 patients were in remission, one had a partial response and one patient did not respond at all [182]. In one study comparing adjunctive IA versus Rituximab therapy, antibody levels, clinical improvement as assessed by the Autoimmune Bullous Skin Disorder Intensity Score (ABSIS) and oral steroid doses all reduced faster in the IA group compared to the Rituximab group. However, there were more relapses in the IA group requiring further treatment [183].

Despite the evidence for IA in PV, an autoimmune disease with well-defined pathogenic IgG autoantibodies, its widespread adoption has been limited. This has been hampered by the small study numbers, lack of RCTs and multiple treatment protocols. Given this PV is a recommended indication for the use of IA by the ASFA where it is classified as a category III disease (optimum role of apheresis therapy is not established) with 2C evidence (weak recommendation, low-quality or very low-quality evidence) [98]. The British Association of

Dermatologists guidelines for the treatment of pemphigus vulgaris also state that IA could be considered in patients unresponsive or intolerant to standard treatment [174].

5.4.2. *Bullous pemphigoid*

Bullous pemphigoid (BP) is an autoimmune condition resulting in the development of subepidermal blisters or bullae and is the most common of the autoimmune blistering conditions. It is caused by IgG autoantibodies directed against the BP180 and the BP230 antigens found in the hemidesmosomes. The mainstay of treatment is the use of topical or systemic steroids with or without oral immunosuppression [184, 185]. In patients refractory to this, IA has been used with varying success.

Herrero-González et al. used tryptophan IA to treat two patients with BP initially unresponsive to methylprednisolone, dapsone and in one patient, additional azathioprine and topical clobetasol propionate. Both patients saw dramatic improvement in their skin lesions after 2 weeks with all active lesions disappearing by 6 weeks [186]. Kasperkiewicz et al. treated seven patients with severe disease using protein A immunoadsorption. Here four patients had previously failed treatment with oral steroids, topical clobetasol propionate and either dapsone or mycophenolate mofetil and three were immunosuppression naïve. All patients saw a significant reduction in circulating antibodies and had no active lesions 1–3 months after therapy. Six of the seven patients remained in clinical remission at the end of follow up with two of the patients requiring no adjuvant medication [187]. Ino et al. used dextran sulfate conjugated cellulose columns to treat two patients who had not responded to steroids or dapsone. In one patient the lesions disappeared 2 weeks after treatment however in the second patient the skin lesions returned after 6 weeks and despite a second course of IA continued to have active blistering [188].

Given the pathogenicity of the IgG antibodies involved in BP and the positive results, albeit from very limited published data, IA has the potential to provide adjunctive therapy in refractory BP.

5.4.3. *Atopic dermatitis*

Atopic dermatitis (AD) is a chronic inflammatory condition affecting up to 20% of the population [189]. It is characterised by recurrent pruritic eczematous lesions and generally presents in childhood. Its pathogenesis is not completely understood, exacerbated by the heterogeneous nature of the disease, but genetic, environmental and humoral factors are all associated with its development. The disease itself can be associated with other atopic and inflammatory conditions such as asthma, allergic rhinitis and inflammatory bowel disease. Far from being a typical type I hypersensitivity reaction as initially thought it now appears to be a complex combination of epidermal barrier dysfunction, T helper 2 (Th2) cell-mediated and IgE immune regulated pathways. The majority of patients show a raised serum IgE titre with some circumstantial evidence suggesting it plays a pathogenic role [190, 191].

The first published study used IA in 12 patients with severe AD and total serum IgE levels of >4500 kU/L. Patients saw a significant improvement in their mean Scoring Atopic Dermatitis

(SCORAD), reducing from 78.6 ± 3.9 to 32.4 ± 3.5 at the end of the study at week 13. There were also significant improvements seen in the mean Eczema Area and Severity Index (EASI) and the pruritus score by the end of the study [192]. Since that time there has been a large number of patients treated in clinical trials with promising results [193–196]. Reich et al. treated 26 severe AD patients with IgE specific IA and 24 patients with a Pan-immunoglobulin IA. Both groups reported an equal improvement in their EASI scores with almost 50% of patients reporting a >50% improvement. There were also improvements seen in the Dermatology Life Quality Index (DLQI), the SCORAD and the Patient-Oriented Eczema Measure (POEM). In this study the IgE specific adsorber was better tolerated with less adverse events than the pan-immunoglobulin adsorber with similar clinical outcomes [196].

Given the weight of evidence now accumulating and the safety profile of the IgE specific adsorbers, IA should be considered in the case of AD unresponsive to standard care or in those in whom it is contraindicated.

5.5. Respiratory

5.5.1. Asthma

Asthma is one of the world's most prevalent chronic diseases affecting an estimated 300 million people worldwide and rising. A variant of asthma, allergic asthma is classified as a type 1 hypersensitivity reaction. Here IgE binds to high-affinity FcεRI receptors on Mast cells and Basophils leading to degranulation and the release of inflammatory mediators. There is now increasing evidence that the incidence of IgE-mediated allergies is on the rise. In allergic asthma, as in other allergen related disease, the severity is progressive as patients come into contact with the allergen over time [197–199].

The IgEnio is a single use IgE specific adsorber developed by Fresenius Medical Care. The ESPIRA trial (Extracorporeal IgE Immunoadsorption in Allergic Asthma: Safety and Efficacy) is a randomized controlled trial investigating the efficacy of IA in 14 adult patients with allergic asthma and raised IgE titres. Patients were treated for three cycles with each cycle consisting of three sessions. Mean IgE levels reduced by 87% per cycle for total IgE with similar reductions in IgE specific for seasonal and perennial allergens. A steady improvement in peak flow levels, overall allergy symptoms as assessed by the Visual Analogue Scale (VAS) and lung specific symptoms were also seen. In the US, omalizumab is only indicated in patients with an IgE titre of below 700 U/ml and in the EU below 1500 U/ml. Along with the clinical and biochemical improvements seen with the treatment, interestingly it also allowed three of the patients, who were previously ineligible for omalizumab due to their high titres, to qualify for omalizumab treatment. Further work is needed given this is the first reported use of IA in allergic asthma but the initial findings are promising [199].

6. Conclusion

Despite recent healthcare advances, sepsis remains a significant cause of morbidity, mortality and admission to ICU. However, new technologies with the ability to remove damaging factors

http://dx.doi.org/10.5772/intechopen.84890

in the pathogenesis of sepsis may help to improve patient outcomes. Since its development over 2 decades ago, immunoadsorption therapy has proven to be a highly efficient method of removing antibodies with a remarkably safe side effect profile. As our understanding of not only sepsis but also autoimmune disease increases, the range of conditions that are amenable to IA will also increase. With the development of columns for more specific antibodies and molecules such as those for sepsis, its use can reasonably be expected to become more ubiquitous.

Acknowledgements

This work is supported by the National Institute of Health Research (NIHR) Devices for Dignity Med tech Co-operative (D4D). The views expressed are those of the authors and not necessarily those of the NHS, the NIHR or the Department of Health.

Author details

Patrick Hamilton[1,2], Rhodri Harris[1] and Sandip Mitra[2,3]*

*Address all correspondence to: sandip.mitra@cmft.nhs.uk

1 Manchester Royal Infirmary, Manchester, United Kingdom

2 Manchester Academic Health Science Centre (MAHSC), The University of Manchester, Manchester, United Kingdom

3 NIHR Devices for Dignity, MedTech Co-operative, Manchester, United Kingdom

References

[1] Gjörstrup P. Therapeutic protein A immunoadsorption. A review. Transfusion Science. 1990;**11**(3):281-302

[2] Rönspeck W, Brinckmann R, Egner R, Gebauer F, Winkler D, Jekow P, et al. Peptide based adsorbers for therapeutic immunoadsorption. Therapeutic Apheresis and Dialysis. 2003;**7**(1):91-97

[3] Kaplan AA. A simple and accurate method for prescribing plasma exchange. ASAIO Transactions. 1990;**36**(3):M597-M599

[4] Tsuboi Y, Takahashi M, Ishikawa Y, Okada H, Yamada T. Elevated bradykinin and decreased carboxypeptidase R as a cause of hypotension during tryptophan column immunoabsorption therapy. Therapeutic Apheresis. 1998;**2**(4):297-299

[5] Singer M, Deutschman CS, Seymour CW, Shankar-Hari M, Annane D, Bauer M, et al. The third international consensus definitions for sepsis and septic shock (Sepsis-3). Journal of the American Medical Association. 2016;**315**(8):801-810

[6] van Gestel A, Bakker J, Veraart CP, van Hout BA. Prevalence and incidence of severe sepsis in Dutch intensive care units. Critical Care. 2004;**8**(4):153-162

[7] Fullerton JN, Thompson K, Shetty A, Iredell JR, Lander H, Myburgh JA, et al. New sepsis definition changes incidence of sepsis in the intensive care unit. Critical Care and Resuscitation. 2017;**19**(1):9-13

[8] Gotts JE, Matthay MA. Sepsis: Pathophysiology and clinical management. British Medical Journal. 2016:i1585-i1520

[9] Angus DC, van der Poll T. Severe sepsis and septic shock. The New England Journal of Medicine. 2013;**369**(9):840-851

[10] Schrier RW, Wang W. Acute renal failure and sepsis. The New England Journal of Medicine. 2004;**351**(2):159-169

[11] Kumar A, Roberts D, Wood KE, Light B, Parrillo JE, Sharma S, et al. Duration of hypotension before initiation of effective antimicrobial therapy is the critical determinant of survival in human septic shock. Critical Care Medicine. 2006;**34**(6):1589-1596

[12] Venkatesh B, Finfer S, Cohen J, Rajbhandari D, Arabi Y, Bellomo R, et al. Adjunctive glucocorticoid therapy in patients with septic shock. The New England Journal of Medicine. 2018;**378**(9):797-808

[13] Annane D, Renault A, Brun-Buisson C, Megarbane B, Quenot J-P, Siami S, et al. Hydrocortisone plus fludrocortisone for adults with septic shock. The New England Journal of Medicine. 2018;**378**(9):809-818

[14] Suffredini AF. A role for hydrocortisone therapy in septic shock? The New England Journal of Medicine. 2018;**378**(9):860-861

[15] Toussaint S, Gerlach H. Activated protein C for sepsis. The New England Journal of Medicine. 2009;**361**(27):2646-2652

[16] Ranieri VM, Thompson BT, Barie PS, Dhainaut J-F, Douglas IS, Finfer S, et al. Drotrecogin alfa (activated) in adults with septic shock. The New England Journal of Medicine. 2012; **366**(22):2055-2064

[17] Fujii T, Ganeko R, Kataoka Y, Furukawa TA, Featherstone R, Doi K, et al. Polymyxin B-immobilized hemoperfusion and mortality in critically ill adult patients with sepsis/ septic shock: A systematic review with meta-analysis and trial sequential analysis. Intensive Care Medicine. 2017;**44**(2):167-178

[18] Abstracts of the 33rd International Symposium on Intensive Care and Emergency Medicine. Brussels, Belgium. March 19-22, 2013. Critical Care (London, England). 2013; **17**(Suppl 2):545

[19] National Institute for Health. CytoSorb therapy for Sepsis [Internet]. 2016. Available from: nice.org.uk/guidance/mib87 [Accessed: 29 January 2019]

[20] Malard B, Lambert C, Kellum JA. *In vitro* comparison of the adsorption of inflammatory mediators by blood purification devices. Intensive Care Medicine Experimental. 2018 May 4;**6**(1):12. DOI: 10.1186/s40635-018-0177-2

[21] Schefold JC, Haehling von S, Corsepius M, Pohle C, Kruschke P, Zuckermann H, et al. A novel selective extracorporeal intervention in sepsis: Immunoadsorption of endotoxin, interleukin 6, and complement-activating product 5a. Shock. 2007;**28**(4):418-425

[22] Wyld M, Morton RL, Hayen A, Howard K, Webster AC. A Systematic review and meta-analysis of utility-based quality of life in chronic kidney disease treatments. Turner N, editor. PLoS Medicine. 2012;**9**(9):e1001307-e1001310

[23] Overbeck I, Bartels M, Decker O, Harms J. Changes in quality of life after renal transplantation. Transplantation. Transplant Proceedings. 2005 Apr;**37**(3):1618-1621

[24] Schnuelle P, Lorenz D, Trede M, van der Woude FJ. Impact of renal cadaveric transplantation on survival in end-stage renal failure: Evidence for reduced mortality risk compared with hemodialysis during long-term follow-up. Journal of the American Society of Nephrology. 1998;**9**(11):2135-2141

[25] Organ Donation and Transplantation Activity report 2017/18 [Internet]. 2018. pp. 1-166. Available from: https://nhsbtdbe.blob.core.windows.net/umbraco-assets/1848/transplant-activity-report-2017-2018.pdf [Accessed: 27 June 2018]

[26] Morath C, Zeier M, Döhler B, Opelz G, Süsal C. ABO-incompatible kidney transplantation. Frontiers in Immunology. 2017;**8**(2):327-327

[27] Rydberg L. ABO-incompatibility in solid organ transplantation. Transfusion Medicine. Wiley/Blackwell (10.1111). 2001;**11**(4):325-342

[28] Hume DM, Merrill JP, Miller BF, Thorn GW. Experiences with renal homotransplantation in the human: Report of nine cases. The Journal of clinical investigation. American Society for Clinical Investigation. 1955;**34**(2):327-382

[29] Dunea G, Nakamoto S, Straffon RA, Figueroa JE, Versaci AA, Shibagaki M, et al. Renal homotransplantation in 24 patients. British Medical Journal. 1965;**1**(5426):7-13

[30] Starzl TE, Tzakis A, Makowka L, Banner B, Demetrius A, Ramsey G, et al. The definition of ABO factors in transplantation: Relation to other humoral antibody states. Transplantation Proceedings. 1987;**19**(6):4492-4497

[31] Landsteiner K. Uber Agglutinationserscheinungen normalen menschlichen Blutes. Wiener klinische Wochenschrift. 1901;**14**:1132-1134

[32] Milland J, Sandrin MS. ABO blood group and related antigens, natural antibodies and transplantation. Tissue Antigens. 2006;**68**(6):459-466

[33] Tydén G, Donauer J, Wadström J, Kumlien G, Wilpert J, Nilsson T, et al. Implementation of a protocol for ABO-incompatible kidney transplantation—A three-center experience with 60 consecutive transplantations. Transplantation. 2007 May 15;**83**(9):1153-1155

[34] Tydén G, Kumlien G, Genberg H, Sandberg J, Lundgren T, Fehrman I. ABO incompatible kidney transplantations without splenectomy, using antigen-specific immunoadsorption and rituximab. American Journal of Transplantation. 2005;**5**(1):145-148

[35] Genberg H, Kumlien G, Wennberg L, Tydén G. Long-Term Results of ABO-Incompatible Kidney Transplantation with Antigen-Specific Immunoadsorption and Rituximab. Transplantation. **84**(12 suppl):S44-S47

[36] van Agteren M, Weimar W, de Weerd AE, te Boekhorst PA, Ijzermans JN, van de Wetering J, et al. The first fifty ABO blood group incompatible kidney transplantations: The Rotterdam experience. Journal of Transplantation. 2014;**2014**(11):1-6

[37] Wilpert J, Fischer KG, Pisarski P, Wiech T, Daskalakis M, Ziegler A, et al. Long-term outcome of ABO-incompatible living donor kidney transplantation based on antigen-specific desensitization. An observational comparative analysis. Nephrology, Dialysis, Transplantation. 2010;**25**(11):3778-3786

[38] Thölking G, Koch R, Pavenstädt H, Schuette-Nuetgen K, Busch V, Wolters H, et al. Antigen-specific versus non-antigen-specific immunoadsorption in ABO-incompatible renal transplantation. Bueno V, editor. PLoS ONE. 2015;**10**(6):e0131465–e0131416

[39] Opelz G, Mytilineos J, Wujciak T, Schwarz V, Study DBFTCT. Current status of HLA matching in renal transplantation. The Clinical Investigator. 1992;**70**(9):767-772

[40] Opelz G, Wujciak T, Döhler B, Scherer S, Mytilineos J. HLA compatibility and organ transplant survival. Collaborative transplant Study. Reviews in Immunogenetics. 1999; **1**(3):334-342

[41] Hyun J, Park KD, Yoo Y, Lee B. Effects of different sensitization events on HLA alloimmunization in solid organ transplantation patients. Transplantation Proceedings. 2012;**44**(1):222-225

[42] Yabu JM, Anderson MW, Kim D, Bradbury BD, Lou CD, Petersen J, et al. Sensitization from transfusion in patients awaiting primary kidney transplant. Nephrology, Dialysis, Transplantation. 2013;**28**(11):2908-2918

[43] Hickey MJ, Valenzuela NM, Reed EF. Alloantibody generation and effector function following sensitization to human leukocyte antigen. Frontiers in Immunology. 2016;**7**(2):699

[44] Regan L, Braude PR, Hill DP. A prospective study of the incidence, time of appearance and significance of anti-paternal lymphocytotoxic antibodies in human pregnancy. Human Reproduction. 1991;**6**(2):294-298

[45] Montgomery RA, Lonze BE, King KE, Kraus ES, Kucirka LM, Locke JE, et al. Desensitization in HLA-incompatible kidney recipients and survival. The New England Journal of Medicine. 2011;**365**(4):318-326

[46] Higgins RM, Bevan DJ, Carey BS, Lea CK, Fallon M, Bühler R, et al. Prevention of hyperacute rejection by removal of antibodies to HLA immediately before renal transplantation. Lancet. 1996;**348**(9036):1208-1211

[47] Rostaing L, Congy N, Aarnink A, Maggioni S, Allal A, Sallusto F, et al. Efficacy of immunoadsorption to reduce donor-specific alloantibodies in kidney-transplant candidates. Experimental and Clinical Transplantation. 2015;**13**(Suppl 1):201-206

[48] Lorenz M, Regele H, Schillinger M, Kletzmayr J, Haidbauer B, Derfler K, et al. Peritransplant immunoadsorption: A strategy enabling transplantation in highly sensitized crossmatch-positive cadaveric kidney allograft recipients. Transplantation. 2005; **79**(6):696-701

[49] Rivera F, López-Gómez JM, Pérez-García R, Spanish Registry of Glomerulonephritis. Frequency of renal pathology in Spain 1994-1999. Nephrology, Dialysis, Transplantation. 2002;**17**(9):1594-1602

[50] Braden GL, Mulhern JG, O'Shea MH, Nash SV, Ucci AA Jr, Germain MJ. Changing incidence of glomerular diseases in adults. American Journal of Kidney Diseases. 2000; **35**(5):878-883

[51] Swaminathan S, Leung N, Lager DJ, Melton LJ, Bergstralh EJ, Rohlinger A, et al. Changing incidence of glomerular disease in Olmsted County, Minnesota: A 30-year renal biopsy study. Clinical Journal of the American Society of Nephrology. 2006;**1**(3): 483-487

[52] Simon P, Ramee M-P, Boulahrouz R, Stanescu C, Charasse C, Ang KS, et al. Epidemiologic data of primary glomerular diseases in western France. Kidney International. 2004; **66**(3):905-908

[53] Malafronte P, Mastroianni-Kirsztajn G, Betônico GN, João Egídio Romão J, MAR A, Carvalho MF, et al. Paulista registry of glomerulonephritis: 5-year data report. Nephrology, Dialysis, Transplantation. 2006;**21**(11):3098-3105

[54] McGrogan A, Franssen CFM, de Vries CS. The incidence of primary glomerulonephritis worldwide: A systematic review of the literature. Nephrology, Dialysis, Transplantation. 2011;**26**(2):414-430

[55] Beck LH Jr, Bonegio RGB, Lambeau G, Beck DM, Powell DW, Cummins TD, et al. M-type phospholipase A2 Receptor as target antigen in idiopathic membranous nephropathy. The New England Journal of Medicine. 2009;**361**(1):11-21

[56] Ponticelli C, Zucchelli P, Passerini P, Cesana B, Locatelli F, Pasquali S, et al. A 10-year follow-up of a randomized study with methylprednisolone and chlorambucil in membranous nephropathy. Kidney International. 1995;**48**(5):1600-1604

[57] Ponticelli C, Altieri P, Scolari F, Passerini P, Roccatello D, Cesana B, et al. A randomized study comparing methylprednisolone plus chlorambucil versus methylprednisolone plus cyclophosphamide in idiopathic membranous nephropathy. Journal of the American Society of Nephrology. 1998;**9**(3):444-450

[58] Eknoyan G, Eckardt KU, Kasiske BL. KDIGO clinical practice guideline for glomerulonephritis. Kidney International. 2012;**2**:143

[59] Kanigicherla D, Gummadova J, McKenzie EA, Roberts SA, Harris S, Nikam M, et al. Anti-PLA2R antibodies measured by ELISA predict long-term outcome in a prevalent population of patients with idiopathic membranous nephropathy. Kidney International. 2013;**83**(5):940-948

[60] Hoxha E, Thiele I, Zahner G, Panzer U, Harendza S, Stahl RAK. Phospholipase A2 receptor autoantibodies and clinical outcome in patients with primary membranous nephropathy. Journal of the American Society of Nephrology. 2014;**25**(6):1357-1366

[61] Beck LH, Fervenza FC, Beck DM, Bonegio RGB, Malik FA, Erickson SB, et al. Rituximab-induced depletion of anti-PLA2R autoantibodies predicts response in membranous nephropathy. Journal of the American Society of Nephrology. 2011;**22**(8):1543-1550

[62] Ruggenenti P, Debiec H, Ruggiero B, Chianca A, Pellé T, Gaspari F, et al. Anti-phospholipase A2 receptor antibody Titer predicts post-rituximab outcome of membranous nephropathy. Journal of the American Society of Nephrology. 2015;**26**(10): 2545-2558

[63] Esnault VL, Besnier D, Testa A, Coville P, Simon P, Subra JF, et al. Effect of protein a immunoadsorption in nephrotic syndrome of various etiologies. Journal of the American Society of Nephrology. 1999;**10**(9):2014-2017

[64] Hamilton P, Kanigicherla D, Hanumapura P, Walz L, Kramer D, Fischer M, et al. Peptide GAM immunoadsorption therapy in primary membranous nephropathy (PRISM): Phase II trial investigating the safety and feasibility of peptide GAM immunoadsorption in anti-PLA 2R positive primary membranous nephropathy. Journal of Clinical Apheresis. 2017;**17**(9):1594-1598

[65] Salama AD, Levy JB, Lightstone L, Pusey CD. Goodpasture's disease. Lancet. 2001; **358**(9285):917-920

[66] Merkel F, Pullig O, Marx M, Netzer KO, Weber M. Course and prognosis of anti-basement membrane antibody (anti-BM-Ab)-mediated disease: Report of 35 cases. Nephrology, Dialysis, Transplantation. 1994;**9**(4):372-376

[67] Lockwood CM, Pearson TA, Rees AJ, Evans D, Peters DK, Wilson CB. Immunosuppression and plasma-exchange in the treatment of Goodpasture's syndrome. Immunobiology. 1976;**1**(7962):711-715

[68] Lerner RA, Glassock RJ, Dixon FJ. The role of anti-glomerular basement membrane antibody in the pathogenesis of human glomerulonephritis. The Journal of Experimental Medicine. 1967;**126**(6):989-1004

[69] Bygren P, Freiburghaus C, Lindholm T, Simonsen O, Thysell H, Wieslander J. Goodpasture's syndrome treated with staphylococcal protein a immunoadsorption. Lancet. 1985;**2**(8467):1295-1296

[70] Hu W, Liu Z, Ji D, Xie H, Gong D, Li L. Staphylococcal protein a immunoadsorption for Goodpasture's syndrome in four Chinese patients. Journal of Nephrology. 2006;**19**(3): 312-317

[71] Esnault VLM, Testa A, Jayne DRW, Soulillou JP, Guenel J. Influence of immunoadsorption on the removal of immunoglobulin G autoantibodies in crescentic glomerulonephritis. Nephron. 1993;**65**(2):180-184

[72] Moreso F, Poveda R, Gil-Vernet S, Carreras L, García-Osuna R, Griñó JM, et al. Therapeutic immunoadsorption in Goodpasture disease. Medicina Clínica (Barcelona). 1995;**105**(2):59-61

[73] Stegmayr BG, Almroth G, Berlin G, Fehrman I, Kurkus J, Norda R, et al. Plasma exchange or immunoadsorption in patients with rapidly progressive crescentic glomerulonephritis. A Swedish multi-center study. The International Journal of Artificial Organs. 1999;**22**(2):81-87

[74] Laczika K, Knapp S, Derfler K, Soleiman A, Hörl WH, Druml W. Immunoadsorption in Goodpasture's syndrome. American Journal of Kidney Diseases. 2000;**36**(2):392-395

[75] Biesenbach P, Kain R, Derfler K, Perkmann T, Soleiman A, Benharkou A, et al. Long-term outcome of anti-glomerular basement membrane antibody disease treated with immunoadsorption. PLoS One. 2014;**9**(7):e103568

[76] Appel GB, Contreras G, Dooley MA, Ginzler EM, Isenberg D, Jayne D, et al. Mycophenolate mofetil versus cyclophosphamide for induction treatment of lupus nephritis. Journal of the American Society of Nephrology. 2009;**20**(5):1103-1112

[77] Sawalha AH, Harley JB. Antinuclear autoantibodies in systemic lupus erythematosus. Current Opinion in Rheumatology. 2004;**16**(5):534-540

[78] Malik S, Bruner GR, Williams-Weese C, Feo L, Scofield RH, Reichlin M, et al. Presence of anti-La autoantibody is associated with a lower risk of nephritis and seizures in lupus patients. Lupus. 2007;**16**(11):863-866

[79] Reichlin M. Immunology MW-RC, 2003. Correlations of anti-dsDNA and anti-ribosomal P autoantibodies with lupus nephritis. Immunobiology. 2003;**108**(1):69-72

[80] Biesenbach P, Derfler K, Smolen J, Stummvoll G. THU0282 immunoadsorption in lupus nephritis: Three different high affinity columns are equally effective in inducing remission. Annals of the Rheumatic Diseases. 2013;**72**(Suppl 3):A261

[81] Suzuki K. The role of immunoadsorption using dextran-sulfate cellulose columns in the treatment of systemic lupus erythematosus. Therapeutic Apheresis. 2000;**4**(3):239-243

[82] Gaubitz M, Seidel M, Kummer S, Schotte H, Perniok A, Domschke W, et al. Prospective randomized trial of two different immunoadsorbers in severe systemic lupus erythematosus. Journal of Autoimmunity. 1998;**11**(5):495-501

[83] Stummvoll GH. IgG immunoadsorption reduces systemic lupus erythematosus activity and proteinuria: A long-term observational study. Annals of the Rheumatic Diseases. 2005;**64**(7):1015-1021

[84] Stummvoll GH. Immunoadsorption (IAS) for systemic lupus erythematosus. Lupus. 2011;**20**(2):115-119

[85] Stummvoll GH, Schmaldienst S, Smolen JS, Derfler K, Biesenbach P. Lupus nephritis: Prolonged immunoadsorption (IAS) reduces proteinuria and stabilizes global disease activity. Nephrology, Dialysis, Transplantation. 2012;**27**(2):618-626

[86] Schneider M, Berning T, Waldendorf M, Glaser J, Gerlach U. Immunoadsorbent plasma perfusion in patients with systemic lupus erythematosus. The Journal of Rheumatology. 1990;**17**(7):900-907

[87] Bombardier C, Gladman DD, Urowitz MB, Caron D, Chang CH, Austin A, et al. Derivation of the sledai. A disease activity index for lupus patients. Arthritis and Rheumatism. 1992; **35**(6):630-640

[88] Liang MH, Socher SA, Larson MG, Schur PH. Reliability and validity of six systems for the clinical assessment of disease activity in systemic lupus erythematosus. Arthritis and Rheumatism. 1989;**32**(9):1107-1118

[89] Yu C, Yen TS, Lowell CA, DeFranco AL. Lupus-like kidney disease in mice deficient in the Src family tyrosine kinases Lyn and Fyn. Current Biology. 2001;**11**(1):34-38

[90] Sim JJ, Batech M, Hever A, Harrison TN, Avelar T, Kanter MH, et al. Distribution of biopsy-proven presumed primary glomerulonephropathies in 2000-2011 among a racially and ethnically diverse US population. American Journal of Kidney Diseases. 2016;**68**(4):533-544

[91] Rosenberg AZ, Kopp JB. Focal segmental glomerulosclerosis. Clinical Journal of the American Society of Nephrology. 2017;**12**(3):502-517

[92] Königshausen E, Sellin L. Circulating permeability factors in primary focal segmental glomerulosclerosis: A Review of proposed candidates. BioMed Research International. 2016;**2016**(4):1-9

[93] Haas M, Godfrin Y, Oberbauer R, Yilmaz N, Borchhardt K, Regele H, et al. Plasma immunadsorption treatment in patients with primary focal and segmental glomerulosclerosis. Nephrology, Dialysis, Transplantation. 1998;**13**(8):2013-2016

[94] Martin-Moreno PL, Rifon J, Errasti P. Efficacy of the combination of immunoadsorption and rituximab for treatment in a case of severe focal and segmental glomerulosclerosis recurrence after renal transplantation. Blood Purification. 2018;**46**(2):90-93

[95] Yokoyama K, Sakai S, Sigematsu T, Takemoto F, Hara S, Yamada A, et al. LDL adsorption improves the response of focal glomerulosclerosis to corticosteroid therapy. Clinical Nephrology. 1998;**50**(1):1-7

[96] Muso E, Mune M, Yorioka N, Nishizawa Y, Hirano T, Hattori M, et al. Beneficial effect of low-density lipoprotein apheresis (LDL-A) on refractory nephrotic syndrome (NS) due to focal glomerulosclerosis (FGS). Clinical Nephrology. 2007;**67**(6):341-344

[97] Muso E, Mune M, Fujii Y, Imai E, Ueda N, Hatta K, et al. Significantly rapid relief from steroid-resistant nephrotic syndrome by LDL apheresis compared with steroid monotherapy. Nephron. 2001;**89**(4):408-415

[98] Schwartz J, Padmanabhan A, Aqui N, Balogun RA, Connelly-Smith L, Delaney M, et al. Guidelines on the use of therapeutic apheresis in clinical practice-evidence-based approach from the writing Committee of the American Society for apheresis: The seventh special issue. Journal of Clinical Apheresis. 2016;**31**(3):149-338

[99] Jennette JC, Nachman PH. ANCA glomerulonephritis and vasculitis. Clinical Journal of the American Society of Nephrology. 2017;**12**(10):1680-1691

[100] Seo P, Stone JH. The antineutrophil cytoplasmic antibody—Associated vasculitides. The American Journal of Medicine. 2004;**117**(1):39-50

[101] Walton EW. Giant-cell granuloma of the respiratory tract (Wegener's granulomatosis). British Medical Journal. 1958;**2**(5091):265-270

[102] Walsh M, Merkel PA, Peh CA, Szpirt W, Guillevin L, Pusey CD, et al. Plasma exchange and glucocorticoid dosing in the treatment of anti-neutrophil cytoplasm antibody associated vasculitis (PEXIVAS): Protocol for a randomized controlled trial. Trials. 2013;**14**(1):73

[103] Flossmann O, Berden A, De Groot K, Hagen C, Harper L, Heijl C, et al. Long-term patient survival in ANCA-associated vasculitis. Annals of the Rheumatic Diseases. 2011;**70**(3):488-494

[104] Seo P, Min YI, Holbrook JT, Hoffman GS, Merkel PA, Spiera R, et al. Damage caused by Wegener's granulomatosis and its treatment: Prospective data from the Wegener's granulomatosis etanercept trial (WGET). Arthritis and Rheumatism. 2005;**52**(7):2168-2178

[105] Hoffman GS, Kerr GS, Leavitt RY, Hallahan CW, Lebovics RS, Travis WD, et al. Wegener granulomatosis: An analysis of 158 patients. Annals of Internal Medicine. 1992;**116**(6):488-498

[106] Little MA, Nightingale P, Verburgh CA, Hauser T, De Groot K, Savage C, et al. Early mortality in systemic vasculitis: Relative contribution of adverse events and active vasculitis. Annals of the Rheumatic Diseases. 2010;**69**(6):1036-1043

[107] Porges AJ, Redecha PB, Kimberly WT, Csernok E, Gross WL, Kimberly RP. Anti-neutrophil cytoplasmic antibodies engage and activate human neutrophils via fc gamma RIIa. Journal of Immunology. 1994;**153**(3):1271-1280

[108] Matic G, Michelsen A, Hofmann D, Winkler R, Tiess M, Schneidewind JM, et al. Three cases of C-ANCA-positive Vasculitis treated with immunoadsorption: Possible benefit in early treatment. Therapeutic Apheresis and Dialysis. 2001;**5**(1):68-72

[109] Koch M, Kohnle M, Trapp R. A case report of successful long-term relapse control by protein-a immunoadsorption in an immunosuppressive-treated patient with end-stage renal disease due to Wegener's granulomatosis. Therapeutic Apheresis and Dialysis. 2009;**13**(2):150-156

[110] Danesh J, Collins R, Peto R. Lipoprotein(a) and coronary heart disease: Meta-analysis of prospective studies. Circulation. 2000;**102**(10):1082-1085

[111] Emerging Risk Factors Collaboration, Erqou S, Kaptoge S, Perry PL, Di Angelantonio E, Thompson A, et al. Lipoprotein(a) concentration and the risk of coronary heart disease, stroke, and nonvascular mortality. Journal of the American Medical Association. 2009;**302**(4):412-423

[112] Defesche JC, Gidding SS, Harada-Shiba M, Hegele RA, Santos RD, Wierzbicki AS. Familial hypercholesterolaemia. Nature Reviews. Disease Primers. 2017;**3**:17093

[113] National Institute for Health and Clinical Excellence. Familial hypercholesterolaemia: Identifification and management - clinical guideline (CG71). 2008:1-35

[114] Goldberg AC, Hopkins PN, Toth PP, Ballantyne CM, Rader DJ, Robinson JG, et al. Familial hypercholesterolemia: Screening, diagnosis and management of pediatric and adult patients: Clinical Guidance from the National Lipid Association Expert Panel on Familial Hypercholesterolemia. Journal of Clinical Lipidology. 2011;**5**:S1-S8

[115] Nordestgaard BG, Langsted A. Lipoprotein(a) as a cause of cardiovascular disease: Insights from epidemiology, genetics, and biology. Journal of Lipid Research. 2016;**57**(11): 1953-1975

[116] Weintraub RG, Semsarian C, MacDonald P. Dilated cardiomyopathy. Immunobiology. 2017;**390**(10092):400-414

[117] Elliott P, Andersson B, Arbustini E, Bilinska Z, Cecchi F, Charron P, et al. Classification of the cardiomyopathies: A position statement from the European society of cardiology working group on myocardial and pericardial diseases. European Heart Journal. 2008;**29**(2):270-276

[118] Bornholz B, Roggenbuck D, Jahns R, Boege F. Diagnostic and therapeutic aspects of β1-adrenergic receptor autoantibodies in human heart disease. Autoimmunity Reviews. 2014;**13**(9):954-962

[119] Dandel M, Wallukat G, Potapov E, Immunobiology RH. Role of β1-adrenoceptor autoantibodies in the pathogenesis of dilated cardiomyopathy. Immunobiology. 2012; **217**(5):511-520

[120] Wallukat G, Reinke P, Dörffel WV, Luther HP, Bestvater K, Felix SB, et al. Removal of autoantibodies in dilated cardiomyopathy by immunoadsorption. International Journal of Cardiology. 1996;**54**(2):191-195

[121] Dandel M, Wallukat G, Englert A, Lehmkuhl HB, Knosalla C, Hetzer R. Long-term benefits of immunoadsorption in β1-adrenoceptor autoantibody-positive transplant candidates with dilated cardiomyopathy. European Journal of Heart Failure. 2014;**14**(12): 1374-1388

[122] Ohlow M-A, Brunelli M, Schreiber M, Lauer B. Therapeutic effect of immunoadsorption and subsequent immunoglobulin substitution in patients with dilated cardiomyopathy: Results from the observational prospective Bad Berka registry. Journal of Cardiology. 2017;**69**(2):409-416

[123] Müller J, Wallukat G, Dandel M, Bieda H, Brandes K, Spiegelsberger S, et al. Immunoglobulin adsorption in patients with idiopathic dilated cardiomyopathy. Circulation. 2000;**101**(4):385-391

[124] Felix SB, Staudt A, Landsberger M, Grosse Y, Stangl V, Spielhagen T, et al. Removal of cardiodepressant antibodies in dilated cardiomyopathy by immunoadsorption. Journal of the American College of Cardiology. 2002;**39**(4):646-652

[125] Felix SB, Staudt A, Dörffel WV, Stangl V, Merkel K, Pohl M, et al. Hemodynamic effects of immunoadsorption and subsequent immunoglobulin substitution in dilated cardiomyopathy: Three-month results from a randomized study. Journal of the American College of Cardiology. 2000;**35**(6):1590-1598

[126] Knebel F, Böhm M, Staudt A, Borges AC, Tepper M, Jochmann N, et al. Reduction of morbidity by immunoadsorption therapy in patients with dilated cardiomyopathy. International Journal of Cardiology. 2004;**97**(3):517-520

[127] Doesch AO, Konstandin M, Celik S, Kristen A, Frankenstein L, Hardt S, et al. Effects of protein a immunoadsorption in patients with advanced chronic dilated cardiomyopathy. Journal of Clinical Apheresis. 2009;**24**(4):141-149

[128] Dandel M, Wallukat G, Englert A, Hetzer R. Immunoadsorption therapy for dilated cardiomyopathy and pulmonary arterial hypertension. Atherosclerosis. Supplements. 2013;**14**(1):203-211

[129] Dörffel WV, Felix SB, Wallukat G, Brehme S, Bestvater K, Hofmann T, et al. Short-term hemodynamic effects of immunoadsorption in dilated cardiomyopathy. Circulation. 1997;**95**(8):1994-1997

[130] Cooper LT, Belohlavek M, Korinek J, Yoshifuku S, Sengupta PP, Burgstaler EA, et al. A pilot study to assess the use of protein a immunoadsorption for chronic dilated cardiomyopathy. Journal of Clinical Apheresis. 2007;**22**(4):210-214

[131] Suleiman M, Khatib R, Agmon Y, Mahamid R, Boulos M, Kapeliovich M, et al. Early inflammation and risk of long-term development of heart failure and mortality in survivors of acute myocardial infarction predictive role of C-reactive protein. Journal of the American College of Cardiology. 2006;**47**(5):962-968

[132] Mincu R-I, Jánosi RA, Vinereanu D, Rassaf T, Totzeck M. Preprocedural C-reactive protein predicts outcomes after primary percutaneous coronary intervention in patients with ST-elevation myocardial infarction a systematic meta-analysis. Scientific Reports. 2017;**7**(1):41530

[133] Pepys MB, Hirschfield GM, Tennent GA, Gallimore JR, Kahan MC, Bellotti V, et al. Targeting C-reactive protein for the treatment of cardiovascular disease. Nature. 2006;**440**(7088):1217-1221

[134] Kitsis RN, Jialal I. Limiting myocardial damage during acute myocardial infarction by inhibiting C-reactive protein. The New England Journal of Medicine. 2006;**355**(5):513-515

[135] Sheriff A, Schindler R, Vogt B, Aty HA, Unger JK, Bock C, et al. Selective apheresis of C-reactive protein: A new therapeutic option in myocardial infarction? Journal of Clinical Apheresis. 2015;**30**(1):15-21

[136] Wallukat G, Muñoz Saravia SG, Haberland A, Bartel S, Araujo R, Valda G, et al. Distinct patterns of autoantibodies against G-protein-coupled receptors in Chagas' cardiomyopathy and megacolon. Their potential impact for early risk assessment in asymptomatic Chagas' patients. Journal of the American College of Cardiology. 2010;**55**(5): 463-468

[137] Botoni FA, Ribeiro ALP, Marinho CC, Lima MMO, Nunes MDCP, Rocha MOC. Treatment of Chagas cardiomyopathy. BioMed Research International. 2013;**2013**(6):1-9

[138] Dendrou CA, Fugger L, Friese MA. Immunopathology of multiple sclerosis. 2015; **15**(9):545-558

[139] Reich DS, Lucchinetti CF, Calabresi PA. Multiple sclerosis. The New England Journal of Medicine. 2018;**378**(2):169-180

[140] Thompson AJ, Baranzini SE, Geurts J, Hemmer B, Ciccarelli O. Multiple sclerosis. Lancet. 2018;**391**(10130):1622-1636

[141] GBD 2015 Neurological Disorders Collaborator Group. Global, regional, and national burden of neurological disorders during 1990-2015: A systematic analysis for the Global Burden of Disease Study 2015. Lancet Neurology. 2017;**16**(11):877-897

[142] Miller DH, Leary SM. Primary-progressive multiple sclerosis. Lancet Neurology. 2007 Oct;**6**(10):903-912

[143] Klingel R, Heibges A, Fassbender C. Plasma exchange and immunoadsorption for autoimmune neurologic diseases—Current guidelines and future perspectives. Atherosclerosis. Supplements. 2009;**10**(5):129-132

[144] de Andrés C, Anaya F, Giménez-Roldán S. Plasma immunoadsorption treatment of malignant multiple sclerosis with severe and prolonged relapses. Revista de Neurologia. 2000;**30**(7):601-605

[145] Heigl F, Hettich R, Arendt R, Durner J, Koehler J, Mauch E. Immunoadsorption in steroid-refractory multiple sclerosis: Clinical experience in 60 patients. Atherosclerosis. Supplements. 2013;**14**(1):167-173

[146] Trebst C, Bronzlik P, Kielstein JT, Schmidt BMW, Stangel M. Immunoadsorption therapy for steroid-unresponsive relapses in patients with multiple sclerosis. Blood Purification. 2012;**33**(1-3):1-6

[147] Hosokawa S, Oyamaguchi A, Yoshida O. Successful immunoadsorption with membrane plasmapheresis for multiple sclerosis. ASAIO Transactions. 1989;**35**(3):576-577

[148] Koziolek MJ, Tampe D, Bähr M, Dihazi H, Jung K, Fitzner D, et al. Immunoadsorption therapy in patients with multiple sclerosis with steroid-refractory optical neuritis. Journal of Neuroinflammation. 2012;**9**(1):80

[149] Mühlhausen J, Kitze B, Huppke P, Müller GA, Koziolek MJ. Apheresis in treatment of acute inflammatory demyelinating disorders. Atherosclerosis. Supplements. 2015;**18**(C): 251-256

[150] Willison HJ, Jacobs BC, van Doorn PA. Guillain-Barré syndrome. Lancet. 2016;**388**(10045): 717-727

[151] Rosenow F, Haupt WF, Grieb P, Jiménez-Klingberg C, Borberg H. Plasma exchange and selective adsorption in Guillain-Barré syndrome—A comparison of therapies by clinical course and side effects. Transfusion Science. 1993;**14**(1):13-15

[152] Haupt WF, Rosenow F, van der Ven C, Borberg H, Pawlik G. Sequential treatment of Guillain-Barré syndrome with extracorporeal elimination and intravenous immunoglobulin. Therapeutic Apheresis. 1997;**1**(1):55-57

[153] Marn Pernat A, Buturović-Ponikvar J, Švigelj V, Ponikvar R. Guillain-Barré syndrome treated by membrane plasma exchange and/or immunoadsorption. Therapeutic Apheresis and Dialysis. 2009;**13**(4):310-313

[154] Okamiya S, Ogino M, Ogino Y, Irie S, Kanazawa N, Saito T, et al. Tryptophan-immobilized column-based immunoadsorption as the choice method for plasmapheresis in Guillain-Barré syndrome. Therapeutic Apheresis and Dialysis. 2004;**8**(3):248-253

[155] Dogan Onugoren M, Golombeck KS, Bien C, Abu-Tair M, Brand M, Bulla-Hellwig M, et al. Immunoadsorption therapy in autoimmune encephalitides. Neurology Neuroimmunology and Neuroinflammation. 2016;**3**(2):e207

[156] Köhler W, Ehrlich S, Dohmen C, Haubitz M, Hoffmann F, Schmidt S, et al. Tryptophan immunoadsorption for the treatment of autoimmune encephalitis. European Journal of Neurology. 2015;**22**(1):203-206

[157] Heine J, Ly L-T, Lieker I, Slowinski T, Finke C, Prüss H, et al. Immunoadsorption or plasma exchange in the treatment of autoimmune encephalitis: A pilot study. Journal of Neurology. 2016;**263**(12):2395-2402

[158] Fassbender C, Klingel R, Köhler W. Immunoadsorption for autoimmune encephalitis. Atherosclerosis. Supplements. 2017;**30**:257-263

[159] Mathey EK, Park SB, Hughes RA, Pollard JD, Armati PJ, Barnett MH, et al. Chronic inflammatory demyelinating polyradiculoneuropathy: From pathology to phenotype. Journal of Neurology, Neurosurgery, and Psychiatry. 2015;**86**(9):973-985

[160] Galldiks N, Burghaus L, Dohmen C, Teschner S, Pollok M, Leebmann J, et al. Immunoadsorption in patients with chronic inflammatory demyelinating polyradiculoneuropathy with unsatisfactory response to first-line treatment. European Neurology. 2011;**66**(4):183-189

[161] Zinman LH, Sutton D, Ng E, Nwe P, Ngo M, Bril V. A pilot study to compare the use of the Excorim staphylococcal protein immunoadsorption system and IVIG in chronic inflammatory demyelinating polyneuropathy. Transfusion and Apheresis Science. 2005;**33**(3):317-324

[162] Lieker I, Slowinski T, Harms L, Hahn K, Klehmet J. A prospective study comparing tryptophan immunoadsorption with therapeutic plasma exchange for the treatment of chronic inflammatory demyelinating polyneuropathy. Journal of Clinical Apheresis. 2017;**32**(6):486-493

[163] Karczewski P, Hempel P, Kunze R, Bimmler M. Agonistic autoantibodies to the α(1)-adrenergic receptor and the β(2)-adrenergic receptor in Alzheimer's and vascular dementia. Scandinavian Journal of Immunology. 2012;**75**(5):524-530

[164] Wang J, Ben JG, Masters CL, Wang Y-J. A systemic view of Alzheimer disease—Insights from amyloid-β metabolism beyond the brain. Nature Reviews. Neurology. 2017;**13**(10):612-623

[165] Hempel P, Heinig B, Jerosch C, Decius I, Karczewski P, Kassner U, et al. Immunoadsorption of agonistic autoantibodies against α1-adrenergic receptors in patients with mild to moderate dementia. Therapeutic Apheresis and Dialysis. 2016;**20**(5):523-529

[166] Titulaer MJ, Lang B, Verschuuren JJ. Lambert-Eaton myasthenic syndrome: From clinical characteristics to therapeutic strategies. Lancet Neurology. 2011;**10**(12):1098-1107

[167] Sauter M, Bender A, Heller F, Sitter T. A case report of the efficient reduction of calcium channel antibodies by tryptophan ligand immunoadsorption in a patient with Lambert-Eaton syndrome. Therapeutic Apheresis and Dialysis. 2009;**14**(3):364-367

[168] Baggi F, Ubiali F, Nava S, Nessi V, Andreetta F, Rigamonti A, et al. Effect of IgG immunoadsorption on serum cytokines in MG and LEMS patients. Journal of Neuroimmunology. 2008;**201-202**:104-110

[169] Batchelor TT, Platten M, Hochberg FH. Immunoadsorption therapy for paraneoplastic syndromes. Journal of Neuro-Oncology. 1998;**40**(2):131-136

[170] Ishikawa S, Takei Y, Tokunaga S, Motomura M, Nakao Y, Hanyu N. Response to immunoadsorption and steroid therapies in a patient with carcinomatous Lambert-Eaton myasthenia syndrome accompanied by disturbed consciousness. Rinshō Shinkeigaku. 2000;**40**(5):459-463

[171] Sitaru C, Mihai S, Zillikens D. The relevance of the IgG subclass of autoantibodies for blister induction in autoimmune bullous skin diseases. Archives of Dermatological Research. 2007;**299**(1):1-8

[172] Sharma P, Mao X, Payne AS. Beyond steric hindrance: The role of adhesion signaling pathways in the pathogenesis of pemphigus. Journal of Dermatological Science. 2007;**48**(1):1-14

[173] Payne AS, Hanakawa Y, Amagai M, Stanley JR. Desmosomes and disease: Pemphigus and bullous impetigo. Current Opinion in Cell Biology. 2004;**16**(5):536-543

[174] Harman KE, Brown D, Exton LS, Groves RW, Hampton PJ, Mohd Mustapa MF, et al. British Association of Dermatologists' guidelines for the management of pemphigus vulgaris 2017. The British Journal of Dermatology. 2017;**177**(5):1170-1201

[175] Lüftl M, Stauber A, Mainka A, Klingel R, Schuler G, Hertl M. Successful removal of pathogenic autoantibodies in pemphigus by immunoadsorption with a tryptophan-linked polyvinylalcohol adsorber. The British Journal of Dermatology. 2003;**149**(3):598-605

[176] Schmidt E, Klinker E, Opitz A, Herzog S, Sitaru C, Goebeler M, et al. Protein a immunoadsorption: A novel and effective adjuvant treatment of severe pemphigus. The British Journal of Dermatology. 2003;**148**(6):1222-1229

[177] Shimanovich I, Herzog S, Schmidt E, Opitz A, Klinker E, Bröcker EB, et al. Improved protocol for treatment of pemphigus vulgaris with protein a immunoadsorption. Clinical and Experimental Dermatology. 2006;**31**(6):768-774

[178] Shimanovich I, Nitschke M, Rose C, Grabbe J, Zillikens D. Treatment of severe pemphigus with protein a immunoadsorption, rituximab and intravenous immunoglobulins. The British Journal of Dermatology. 2007;**158**(2):382-388

[179] Frost N, Messer G, Fierlbeck G, Risler T, Lytton SD. Treatment of pemphigus vulgaris with protein a immunoadsorption: Case report of long-term history showing favorable outcome. Annals of the New York Academy of Sciences. 2005;**1051**(1):591-596

[180] Kasperkiewicz M, Shimanovich I, Meier M, Schumacher N, Westermann L, Kramer J, et al. Treatment of severe pemphigus with a combination of immunoadsorption, rituximab, pulsed dexamethasone and azathioprine/mycophenolate mofetil: A pilot study of 23 patients. The British Journal of Dermatology. 2011;**166**(1):154-160

[181] Eming R, Rech J, Barth S, Kalden JR, Schuler G, Harrer T, et al. Prolonged clinical remission of patients with severe pemphigus upon rapid removal of desmoglein-reactive autoantibodies by immunoadsorption. Dermatology. 2006;**212**(2):177-187

[182] Behzad M, Möbs C, Kneisel A, Möller M, Hoyer J, Hertl M, et al. Combined treatment with immunoadsorption and rituximab leads to fast and prolonged clinical remission in difficult-to-treat pemphigus vulgaris. The British Journal of Dermatology. 2012;**166**(4):844-852

[183] Pfütze M, Eming R, Kneisel A, Kuhlmann U, Hoyer J, Hertl M. Clinical and immunological follow-up of pemphigus patients on adjuvant treatment with immunoadsorption or rituximab. Dermatology. 2009;**218**(3):237-245

[184] Bernard P, Antonicelli F. Bullous pemphigoid: A Review of its diagnosis, associations and treatment. American Journal of Clinical Dermatology. 2017;**18**(4):513-528

[185] Schmidt E, Zillikens D. Pemphigoid diseases. Lancet. 2013;**381**(9863):320-332

[186] Herrero-Gonzalez JE, Sitaru C, Klinker E, Bröcker EB, Zillikens D. Successful adjuvant treatment of severe bullous pemphigoid by tryptophan immunoadsorption. Clinical and Experimental Dermatology. 2005;**30**(5):519-522

[187] Kasperkiewicz M, Schulze F, Meier M, van Beek N, Nitschke M, Zillikens D, et al. Treatment of bullous pemphigoid with adjuvant immunoadsorption: A case series. Journal of the American Academy of Dermatology. 2014;**71**(5):1018-1020

[188] Ino N, Kamata N, Matsuura C, Shinkai H, Odaka M. Immunoadsorption for the treatment of bullous pemphigoid. Therapeutic Apheresis. 1997;**1**(4):372-376

[189] Deckers IAG, McLean S, Linssen S, Mommers M, van Schayck CP, Sheikh A. Investigating international time trends in the incidence and prevalence of atopic eczema 1990-2010: A systematic review of epidemiological studies. PLoS One. 2012;**7**(7):e39803

[190] Kasperkiewicz M, Schmidt E, Ludwig RJ, Zillikens D. Targeting IgE antibodies by immunoadsorption in atopic dermatitis. Frontiers in Immunology. 2018;**9**:254

[191] Weidinger S, Beck LA, Bieber T, Kabashima K, Irvine AD. Atopic dermatitis. Nature Reviews. Disease Primers. 2018;**4**(1):1

[192] Kasperkiewicz M, Schmidt E, Frambach Y, Rose C, Meier M, Nitschke M, et al. Improvement of treatment-refractory atopic dermatitis by immunoadsorption: A pilot study. The Journal of Allergy and Clinical Immunology. 2011;**127**(1):267-270.e6

[193] Kasperkiewicz M, Süfke S, Schmidt E, Zillikens D. IgE-specific immunoadsorption for treatment of recalcitrant atopic dermatitis. JAMA Dermatology. 2014;**150**(12):1350-1351

[194] Daeschlein G, Scholz S, Lutze S, Eming R, Arnold A, Haase H, et al. Repetitive immunoadsorption cycles for treatment of severe atopic dermatitis. Therapeutic Apheresis and Dialysis. 2015;**19**(3):279-287

[195] Zink A, Gensbaur A, Zirbs M, Seifert F, Suarez IL, Mourantchanian V, et al. Targeting IgE in severe atopic dermatitis with a combination of immunoadsorption and omalizumab. Acta Dermato-Venereologica. 2016;**96**(1):72-76

[196] Reich K, Deinzer J, Fiege A-K, von Gruben V, Sack A-L, Thraen A, et al. Panimmunoglobulin and IgE-selective extracorporeal immunoadsorption in patients with severe atopic dermatitis. The Journal of Allergy and Clinical Immunology. 2016;**137**(6):1882-1886

[197] Dhami S, Kakourou A, Asamoah F, Agache I, Lau S, Jutel M, et al. Allergen immunotherapy for allergic asthma: A systematic review and meta-analysis. Allergy. 2017;**72**(12):1825-1848

[198] Holgate ST. Innate and adaptive immune responses in asthma. Nature Medicine. 2012; **18**(5):673-683

[199] Lupinek C, Derfler K, Lee S, Prikoszovich T, Movadat O, Wollmann E, et al. Extracorporeal IgE immunoadsorption in allergic asthma: Safety and efficacy. EBioMedicine. 2017 Mar;**17**:119-133. DOI: 10.1016/j.ebiom.2017.02.007

Continuous Renal Replacement Therapy Specialized Teams: A Challenge to Improve Quality Performance

Jorge Echeverri, Carolina Larrarte and
Manuel Huerfano

Additional information is available at the end of the chapter

http://dx.doi.org/10.5772/intechopen.79853

Abstract

Acute kidney injury is a common condition in critical care, and continuous extracorporeal therapies have become part of the requirement for multiorgan support in critically ill patients. Availability of continuous renal replacement therapy (CRRT) in a healthcare center can influence the therapy performance and patient's results, and it is challenging to attain high-quality standards in centers without previous experience in CRRT and with new therapy users. This chapter describes the experience of a highly specialized acute renal care service model with emphasis on timely interventions by an exclusive CRRT team, education and training, protocol development, quality performance improvement, and its impact on optimal clinical and pharmacoeconomic outcomes.

Keywords: renal replacement therapy, acute kidney injury, renal rapid response teams, interprofessional care, multidisciplinary care, patient safety, quality improvement, cost-effectiveness

1. Introduction

Acute kidney injury (AKI) is a clinical syndrome characterized by the abrupt decrease in the glomerular filtration rate (GFR), severe enough to compromise the elimination of waste products and uremic toxins. AKI is common in critically ill patients and has been documented in 30–60% of the hospitalized patients in intensive care unit (ICU) [1]. Its pathophysiology involves complex processes including hemodynamics and inflammation disarrangements, many of which are not entirely understood. AKI has multiple etiologies and clinical manifestations; patients may present a wide spectrum of symptoms ranging from asymptomatic through anuria to multiple organ dysfunctions [2, 3].

Early recognition and timely interventions are important for the prognosis of AKI, as well as controlling associated hospital morbidity and preventing the development of long-term outcomes, such as chronic kidney disease and chronic cardiovascular conditions [4–6]. Approximately 13.3 million cases of AKI are estimated per year worldwide, with 1.7 million attributable deaths and a high health burden associated to the increase of the hospital and ICU length of stay (LOS), days of mechanical ventilation, and dialysis dependence [7].

International registries show that about 13% of ICU patients with AKI may require renal replacement therapies, and the mortality rate in this group could be up to 50% [8, 9]. The high mortality rate in this population reflects the critical state and the development of multiorgan failure. Several years ago, acute renal failure requiring dialysis was one of the most difficult conditions to treat in ICU, especially in patients with hemodynamic instability and risks of tissue hypoperfusion during extracorporeal interventions, due to lack of experience in therapy performing and the side effects related to circuit anticoagulation [10, 11].

The introduction of continuous renal replacement therapy (CRRT) allowed for the possibility of performing safely extracorporeal therapies in ICU, with less specific requirement for dialysis infrastructure and improved medical care in patients with access barriers to dialysis or hemodynamic tolerance concerns [11–13]. From the first continuous arteriovenous hemofiltration, CRRT evolves to veno-venous systems up to the modern integrated full-volume pump monitors, thus becoming a preferred, safe extracorporeal therapy in many critical care patients [14–16].

The success in the implementation of continuous renal replacement therapy (CRRT) in ICU does not depend only on its availability and technological advances, but on the development of excellent programs, where the intervention of specialized doctors and highly trained nurses complement one another. Specialized teams allow for a standardized care with the highest quality safety, facilitating the recognition of specific needs on the critical AKI population, improving decision-making and individualized management. In 1998, Ronco and Bellomo introduced the term "critical nephrology" to highlight the importance of a multidisciplinary approach in the critical patient with AKI, emphasizing the need for training, collaboration, and communication between various clinical teams [17, 18]. Currently, this approach is still valid and the role of the specialized renal care teams becomes relevant [19]. This chapter aims to explain, by means of the experience of a specialized network of critical nephrology teams, the most relevant guidelines in the construction of a rapid renal response team and its expected benefits.

2. Renal emergency team (RET) and a critical nephrology program (CNP): a rationale for critically ill patients

Delay in recognition of serious diseases or their associated complications has been identified in hospital care and ICU as one of the most important factors that could affect clinical outcomes and the consumption of health resources. AKI is a disease with difficult early recognition, high health burden due to its important rate of complications in the short and long term, lack of knowledge of its pathophysiological processes and lack of a specific treatment.

Despite the progress in knowledge achieved in recent years, concerning biomarkers and their incorporation in therapeutic protocols [20, 21], incremental innovations in technology with an emphasis on multi-organic support [22, 23], patients outcomes continue to be suboptimal [24]. AKI is a complex phenomenon that rarely affects only the kidney, it encompasses multiple complex organic dysfunction and alterations in cross-talk between organs [25]; hence, an interdisciplinary approach allows for the knowledge leverage across different specialties. Participation of experts in each area, a specialist in critical nephrology and a highly trained group of CRRT/intermittent hemodialysis (IHD) nurses, potentially helps in priority establishment, implementation of standardized actions, and implementation of quality control processes [26, 27].

Specialized providers external to traditional intensive care staff, but with experience in critically ill patients, is not a recent practice. Areas such as respiratory care practitioners, a nutritional support team, clinical pharmacology, diagnostic and interventional radiology, cardiology, rehabilitation, and physiotherapy are examples of external groups involved in interprofessional care [28]. Requirements of complex patients, incorporation of IT systems and continuous improvement policies, together with advances in health care, are part of the institutional framework necessary to incorporate groups of excellence, facilitate cooperative work, and increase healthcare benefits.

Collaborative work experiences vary between nephrologists and intensivists. Nephrology has maintained leadership in the principles of extracorporeal techniques, while intensive care has deepened multisystemic management of AKI patients. However, at the moment, it is necessary to increase leadership in educational aspects, risk control, and vulnerability management in AKI patients. The critical nephrology team leader works as a medical director and also does clinical follow-up work; medical direction is essential to ensure compliance with the infrastructure, logistics, care staff, diagnostic tools, and treatment and technology standards required for patients. The RET leader manages to engage all the professionals under the same established strategy to overcome the complications associated with AKI and overcome institutional obstacles.

The responsibilities of the critical nephrology team are identification of AKI etiology and severity assessment; AKI prevention strategy; drugs adjustment and identification of nephrotoxins; nutritional prescription adjustment; fluid balance planning and fluid overload monitoring; leadership in the planning, placement, use, and care of vascular access; timing for extracorporeal therapies; strict monitoring during the implementation of the different modalities to ensure compliance with clinical objectives; avoiding dialytrauma; and comprehensive clinical strategy after ICU discharge.

In recent years, there have been some before-after studies documenting the benefits of the interventions performed by a specialized and dedicated CRRT team (SCT) after the implementation of an educational and quality improvement program. Two observational studies in Asia showed that the SCT has a positive impact on outcomes such as improving CRRT filters consumption (42 vs. 23 min, decrease of down time per day (4.8 vs. 3.3 h, $p < 0.001$), fewer days of stay in the ICU (27.5 vs. 21.1d, $p = 0.027$), decrease in red blood cell transfusions (70.7 vs. 63.5%, $p = 0.043$), and improving 90-day survival (29.3 vs. 40.7%, $p = 0.039$) [29, 30].

3. How to implement a CNP and a specialized team: the ARTIST model

After identifying an opportunity to implement a critical nephrology program and consolidate a specialized team, it is essential to develop an integrated care model to meet the fundamental aspects for success in a highly complex system. Below is a description of what we call the ARTIST model:

Alarm systems and risk prediction, **R**eady to evaluate and act, **T**iming **I**nterventions, **S**ystems for quality improvement, **T**ransferring knowledge.

3.1. Alarm systems and risk prediction scores

Early AKI recognition begins with risk stratification in specific populations (cardiovascular surgery, surgery, exposure to contrast media), where easy-to-use risk assessment scales have been developed (**Tables 1–3**). IT systems facilitate the identification of high-risk patients in electronic medical records (EMRs) for the RET to evaluate preventive measures, previous to the exposure, and to plan the follow-up.

Risk factor	Score		
• Hypotension	5		
• Intra-aortic balloon counterpulsation (IABC)	5		
• Congestive heart failure (CHF)	5		
• Age > 75 years	4		
• Anemia	3		
• Diabetes mellitus (DM)	3		
• The volume of contrast media	1 per 100 mL		
Baseline GFR MDRD (mL/min/1.73 m^2)	**Score**		
40–60	2		
20–40	4		
<20	6		
Groups of risk	**Total score**	**CIN risk (%)**	**Dialysis risk (%)**
1	0–5	7.5	0.04
2	6–10	14	0.12
3	11–15	26.1	1.09
4	16 or higher	57.3	12.6

GFR, glomerular filtration rate; MDRD, modification of diet in renal disease equation.

Table 1. Contrast-induced nephropathy (CIN) risk scale [31].

Risk factor		Score
• Female		1
• CHF		1
• LVEF < 35%		1
• IABC		2
• Chronic obstructive pulmonary disease		1
• Diabetes mellitus on insulin		1
• Previous coronary artery bypass grafting (CABG)		1
• Emergent surgery		2
• Valve		1
• Valve + CABG		2
• Another type of surgery		2
• Preoperative creatinine		
1.2–2.1 mg/dL		2
>2.1 mg/dL		5
Risk group	**Total score**	**CSA-AKI risk (%)**
I	0–2	0.4
II	3–5	2
III	6–8	8
IV	9–13	21

CHF: congestive heart failure; LVEF: left ventricular ejection fraction; IABC: intra-aortic balloon counterpulsation.

Table 2. Cardiovascular surgery-associated AKI (CSA-AKI) risk scale [33].

Risk factor (RF)	Groups of risk (n)	P-AKI risk (%)	Hazard ratio (IC)
Age > 56 years			
Male	I (<2RF)	0.2	–
CHF	II (3 RF)	0.8	3.1 (1.9–5.3)
Ascites	III (4RF)	2.0	8.5 (5.3–13.7)
Hypertension	IV (5RF)	3.6	15.4 (9.4–25.2)
Urgent surgery	V (6RF)	9.5	46.2 (26.3–70.9)
Preoperative creatinine >1.2 mg/dL			
DM			

CHF: congestive heart failure.

Table 3. Perioperative-associated AKI risk (P-AKI) scale [37].

The primary prevention activities in AKI include the restriction of identified nephrotoxic agents, prescription of alternatives with lower renal impact, or active renal therapeutic interventions such as nephroprotection protocols for contrast medium or ischemic preconditioning in patients at high risk of CSA-AKI [32].

Sometimes, it is necessary to perform studies with contrast agents in critical patients. It is recommended, as far as possible, to defer exposure in patients with shock or heart failure until the hemodynamic state is restored. Repeated exposure to contrast medium should be avoided. Cases of contrast-induced nephropathy should be postponed for additional exposure to the contrast agent until the glomerular filtration rate (GFR) returns to the baseline.

Several studies have shown that the expansion of intravascular volume and the treatment of dehydration prevent AKI; however, the rate of infusion or the best type of fluid is still unknown [34]. Once the patient is exposed to a toxic agent, it is important to assess the renal injury severity. Controlling AKI-related complications is part of secondary prevention, one common example is fluid overload related to fluid resuscitation in patients with absence of diuresis response [35]. Research on novel AKI biomarkers opens up future possibilities to determine the moment of kidney injury before the GFR impairment. It will be possible to validate the effectiveness of timely medical interventions and potentially control the progression of the AKI in its early phases [36].

However, renal insult is not always possible to anticipate. In recent years, researchers have conducted studies to find scales that involve both preexisting conditions associated with AKI and clinical signs of daily monitoring, such as respiration rate and assessment of consciousness (**Table 4**). The prediction score of acute renal injury (APS) has been validated in the medical and surgical population, reaching a negative predictive value of 94%. Also, patients with APS greater than 5 have a significant increase in the risk of death, 1.9 (CI95 1.1–2.0, $p = 0.015$) [38, 39].

In the pediatric population, other predictive scales of severe AKI have been developed, such as the renal angina index. Recently validated in the adult population, it is a combination of risk conditions and signs of kidney injury; a score greater than 6 has an AUC of 0.76 for the development of severe AKI [40, 41].

Once it is clear how to perform the screening to identify high-risk populations, it is ideal to activate the RET either by healthcare professionals at the bedside, or by electronic alert systems. Several studies have shown that EMR designed to identify patients with AKI and to generate an electronic alert could affect the quality of hospital care, improve the control of this disease, its incidence and progression, and associated complications [42–44].

A critical factor, in keeping the high commitment of the RET in the priority assessment of high-risk patients, is to understand when to trigger the alert and initiate care to avoid phenomena such as habituation and fatigue due to the high workload in low-risk population [45].

3.2. Ready to evaluate and act

Once the alarm system has been defined and the setup criteria determined, a logistical structure must be established considering both human resources and required supplies to guarantee the

Risk factor (RF)	Score			
	0	1	2	3
Age	<60		60–79	≥80
Respiratory rate	<20	≥20		
AVPU (not alert)	Alert			Other
Chronic kidney disease stage 3–5	N	Y		
CHF	N	Y		
DM	N		Y	
Liver disease	N			**Y**
Total APS score	**HA AKI risk (%)**		**Odds ratio (IC)**	
0–3	4		0.4 (0.3–0.5)	
3–4	8		2.2 (1.6–2.9)	
5–6	14		2.3 (1.8–2.9)	
7	28		4.7 (3.1–7.2)	

AVPU: alert, voice, pain, unresponsive scale; CHF: chronic heart failure; DM: diabetes mellitus; Y: Yes; N: No.

Table 4. Acute prediction score (APS) for hospital-acquired (HA) AKI.

level of compliance and a sustainable care system. Rapid response teams should have autonomy and independence regarding budget, staff structure, implementation, and supply chain. Electronic health systems are essential to ensure the traceability of each process and further evaluation of the pharmacoeconomic results, clinical and operational efficiencies obtained by a highly specialized team.

The RET should have a portable module of supplies that could be taken to the bedside, including diagnosis (i.e., point-of-care), tubes for sampling, disposables, personal protection equipment, disinfectants, specific drugs, solutions, vascular assessment (i.e., ultrasound), catheters, and document formats. An additional portable module for patients in renal replacement therapies (RRTs) can include filters, circuits, solutions, quality tests, and the rest of dialysis supplies. The program should simplify the supply chain and inventory control, minimize unnecessary consumption, and optimize administrative processes. Nurses must be empowered in each of these processes [46].

Regarding healthcare staff, the RET must have team players with strong communication skills and a highly ethical commitment. Professionals must comply with training and certifications for AKI risk assessment, comprehensive assessment in intensive care and hospital care patients, monitoring and support in critical conditions, and training for acute extracorporeal renal support techniques [47]. In our institutions, we have managed to consolidate the RET with professionals with either experience in intensive care or trained nurses in dialysis. Training programs for new staff should guarantee a combination of nursing knowledge in both the expertise of primary-secondary-tertiary prevention activities and extracorporeal therapies (**Table 5**).

Clinical training	RRT training
Pathophysiology of acute kidney injury	Acute RRT basic principles and modalities
Risk scales for acute kidney injury and clinical assessment in high-risk patients	Monitors and risk management during acute RRT
How to measure and interpret fluid balance	Dialyzers and set up the circuit
Diagnostics on the AKI patient	Programming and navigation through screens
Primary, secondary and tertiary AKI prevention protocols	Pumps, flows and interpreting pressures during acute RRT
Monitoring systems in the critical patient	Troubleshooting alarms and hands-on skills
Hemodynamic and ventilatory support in the critical patient	Protocols for circuit preservation and identifying the coagulation of the circuit
Best clinical practices in vascular access use and care	Follow-up and EMR; roles and responsibilities; and guidelines and protocols of the program
Infection control	Ethics and compliance

Table 5. Specialized nursing training program.

A specialist in critical nephrology is essential to consolidate the RET. Models with the participation of general practitioners with specific training or residents in nephrology that can support some of the medical care processes may be reasonable depending on the volume and complexity of the care processes, and the academic nature of some institutions. It is essential to guarantee the scope and level of participation in these cases; for actions to be timely executed, the specialist should always participate in the decision-making processes.

The timely involvement of the nephrologist correlates with better outcomes in AKI patients. Soares et al. found in their meta-analysis that the delay in nephrology consultation significantly increases the risk of death with a log OR 0.79 (95CI 0.48–1.1, $p < 0.05$). The log OR controls the overall effect of the sample size, a result greater than 0 represents an increased risk of the measured outcome [48].

The specialist in critical nephrology must know in depth the fundamentals associated with the AKI patient. To understand the context of the critical patient, the specialist should perform a multisystemic approach to be able to align the ICU priorities with AKI interventions. As in the nursing group, the specialist must provide an environment of ongoing dialog and interaction with the ICU consultants, establishing agreements for joint interventions and periodic re-evaluation. Real teamwork between ICU healthcare professionals and the specialized team will enhance the collective learning resulting from the interdisciplinary interaction, improving patient health care [49].

3.3. Timing interventions

Preventive measures would impact the incidence and progression of AKI. The five standards of the AKI bundle are: (1) identify the etiology and try to control it, (2) maintain the best renal protection measures (i.e., mean arterial pressure, glucose control, and euvolemia), (3) avoid new toxicity (contrast agents and daily evaluation for interruption or appropriate adjustment of drugs), (4) evaluate the progression of the injury and control of renal function, and (5) intensify the measures if there is progression. The intensity of invasive monitoring and intervention should be adjusted to multi-organ dysfunction and AKI severity.

The emergence of early AKI biomarkers and the development of AKI care bundles have allowed assessing indirectly feasible interventions that could be done by a specialized team in AKI treatment or prevention. Recently, Kolhe et al. published an analysis of a large match cohort of 3717 patients and found a decreased rate of inhospital death (OR 0.76) and less progression to more severe AKI stage (4.2 vs. 6.7%, $p = 0.02$) in 936 patients (25.6%) who completed the KDIGO care bundle within 24 h of follow-up [50].

Early detection of acute kidney injury by introducing biomarkers with better receiver operating characteristics (ROCs) has begun to change the natural history of the disease. A prospective randomized trial of 121 surgical patients, at high risk of AKI with positive TIMP2-IGBP7, tests the KDIGO care bundle vs. standard care to reduce the incidence of primary AKI. Although they did not reach the primary outcome in the entire population, the subanalysis of the low positive biomarker population (TIMP2-IGBP7: 0.3–2) showed a significant reduction in the incidence of AKI (27 vs. 48%, $p = 0.03$), decrease in moderate and severe AKI (6.7 vs. 19.7%, $p = 0.04$) and shorter duration of hospitalization (16 vs. 21, $p = 0.04$). Furthermore, responders showed a greater reduction in biomarker control levels [21].

In another randomized controlled trial (RCT) in postcardiovascular surgery with a high risk of AKI, 276 patients with positive TIMP2-IGFBP7 were randomized to the KDIGO care bundle vs. standard care. Patients in the intervention group most frequently received inotropic drugs and a vasopressor, tight glucose control, and more often withdrawal of ACEi/ARB. The primary outcome showed a general decrease in the incidence of AKI (55.1 vs. 71%, $p = 0.004$) and less moderate and severe AKI (44.9 vs. 21%, $p = 0.009$) in the intervention group. They did not find differences in the requirement of renal replacement therapies or major adverse kidney events (MAKE) [20].

When medical interventions do not control the progression of the disease or when multisystem involvement is severe, it may be necessary to evaluate the need for extracorporeal renal support. If in doubt, the furosemide stress test can help [51]. At present, the early approach to renal support is widely accepted within the scientific intensive care community, before the deleterious consequences of severe AKI appear [52].

3.4. Systems for quality improvement

During medical interventions, safety and quality have been professional and ethical responsibilities. However, the varied experiences at centers performing CRRT, the lack of evidence proving a protocol better than the others, and the variable needs of critical patients, have resulted in great heterogeneity in practices at the bedside, facilitating the gap between therapeutic intentions and what is achieved. The fragility of the patient in intensive care increases the risk of medical errors, and logistical changes or staff shift in the institutions generates different risk moments during the process of care.

International initiatives have raised the awareness for standardized quality measurements in the care of CRRT in ICU. Identify moments or processes where there are potential interventions, with adequate follow-up is essential to strengthen CRRT programs and evolve towards the practices of centers of excellence. Some examples of activities within a quality improvement program are the continuous evaluation of training and education standards, evaluation of clinical practice guidelines and adherence to protocols, unplanned infield auditing, and team discussion of quality indicators and in-depth analysis of adverse events under different perspectives.

Several quality improvement models have been described and they have in common the identification of an improvement opportunity, the implementation of an action plan, the analysis of the results obtained, and the redefinition of the processes. To do so, it is necessary to have a culture of monitoring and reporting within the work team, i.e., constructive and continuous internal audits in which teams participate proactively and without coercion to achieve professional development and evolution in care processes.

For any center of excellence in CRRT, one must be able to answer correctly three questions: do all patients who benefit from the therapy have access as long as they need it? Is the maintenance of the therapy what we expected? And does the patient receive treatment as medically proposed?

The daily monitoring of CRRTs should include the above questions not only from an opportunity perspective but also from the perspective of team empowerment needed to overcome the obstacles and difficulties. Nursing checklists and internal nursing audits should include CRRT configuration; priming; catheter assessment and care; circuit monitoring; exchange of bags and supplies; troubleshooting and alarm resolution; connection, disconnection, and recirculation; evaluation and early recognition of circuit coagulation; and termination of therapy.

Improving documentation of medical records (EMR) is essential for controlling clinical outcomes, especially if there are special forms in place to monitor treatment. Fluid registration is usually a challenge, but after the personnel overcomes the learning curve, they value the importance of accurate information and optimal fluid management. An excellence center should minimize the risks associated with therapy performance (dialytrauma); the application of checklists (**Table 6**) by nursing coordinators or general practitioners during clinical rounds would allow early interventions and will help to start quality improvement plans in cases of inadequate recognition.

The quality indicators, the results of the internal audits, and the events presented must be analyzed with adequate frequency to achieve compliance with improvement plans. The duration of the circuit, the therapy dose administered, the time of inactivity, and the episodes of bleeding are parameters accepted internationally as quality indicators [53].

3.5. Transferring knowledge

The last part of the care model, and not the least important, is all the activities generated within the team to increase the collective knowledge about managing patients with severe AKI and the activities with the intensive care group to close the interdisciplinary knowledge gaps.

CRRT Patient safety chart

NAME | ID | AGE | APACHE | INITIAL SOFA | ROOM

DIAGNOSIS | RESPONSIBLE | TIME OF CRRT INITIATION | INITIAL FLUID BALANCA

YEAR: ______ MONTH: ________ DAY	1	2	3	4	5	6	7	8	9	10	11	12	13	14	15	16	17	18	19	20	21	22	23	24	25	26	27	28	29	30	31	UTD
1. INFECTION AND ADVERSE EVENTS CONTROL																																TOTAL
Proper cleaning and proper changing of dressing																																
Insertion site without evidence of infection																																
Follow the facility Cleaning & Disinfection protocol																																
Follow the isolation precautions																																
Good vascular access function																																
No ischemic complication associated with access																																
KPI (>80%)																																
2. Adjustment of drugs and toxicity prevention																																
Antibiotics																																
Nephrotoxic have been suspended																																
Vasopressor have been adjusted to the PAM goal																																
Fluid infusion rate meets the goal																																
Phosphate guidelines adopted																																
Potassium guidelines adopted																																
Nutrition guidelines adopted																																
Contrast agent control																																
Best renal protection measures (e.i. glucose control)																																
KPI (>90%)																																
4. CRRT MANAGEMENT																																
Timing intervention																																
Downtime Target < 15%																																
CRRT Deliver dose Target > 25ml/kg/h																																
Filter life time expected																																
Reach ultrafiltration Target > 80%																																
KPI (>80%)																																
5. COMPREHENSIVE INTERVENTIONS																																
Complete EMR																																
Labs test as protocol																																
Measured and control bleeding risk																																
Critically ill rehab guidelines adopted																																
Stress ulcer prophylaxis guidelines adopted																																
DVT prophylaxis guidelines adopted																																
Sedation and analgesia guidelines adopted																																
KPI (>80%)																																
Auditor																																

1	YES		0	NO

Table 6. Patient safety chart.

Discussions of difficult cases, presentations of new scientific literature, and updates of clinical practice guidelines among services are some examples of knowledge transfer activities. Similarly, in the nursing environment, the analysis of quality indicators and opportunities for improvement in patient care constitute feedback and learning activities between the ICU and nephrology nurses.

4. Experience and outcomes of a critical nephrology program and two CRRT specialized teams in a net of an acute service provider in Colombia

The following results are part of an internal audit analyzed by our team from the CNP database in two academic centers in Bogota from 2013 to 2016, where a RET operates CRRT. Renal Therapy Services (RTS) is an external provider of specialized renal care services offering IRRT and CRRT as an ARTIST model to hospitals in Colombia.

4.1. The RTS model

RTS is part of Baxter's renal care division, which provides healthcare services for acute and chronic kidney disease. RTS clinics are located in Latin America, Europe, and Asia, equipped with Baxter technology; RTS is responsible for the supply chain and has the nephrology experts for the management of kidney diseases. Some clinics provide hospital services with specialized clinical staff and critical nephrology training: nephrologists, general practitioners, nurses, and pharmacists. Besides, RTS has centralized management support for the clinical operation, quality assurance and information management, a training-education area, and an IT department. RTS has permanent technical support to guarantee continuous therapy.

RTS together with the hospital clinical staff develops the guidelines for the RET, the triggering process of the RET, and the quality indicators for all the processes involved. RTS is responsible for the specialized team, the timely response, the technology and supplies for the renal intervention.

A key factor identified to enhance opportunity is the close interaction between the hospital staff and the RET. In highly complex institutions with high-risk patients and an important demand for services, it is imperative that the hospital team guarantee cost-effectiveness. The RET leader is the nephrologist, assisted by a nurse who directs and organizes the staff according to the daily requirements of the institution, monitors compliance with the protocols, initiates therapies, evaluates patient safety, and provides continuing education to the staff. When the RET receives an alert, it evaluates the patient and decides whether an intervention is necessary or not. If a patient requires extracorporeal therapy, the nephrologist will choose a modality according to national guidelines. The preferred modality for hemodynamically unstable patients (cardiovascular SOFA 3–4) is CRRT. In these cases, the rest of the RET will join in to generate attention to the patient and prepare all requirements for the vascular access placement and the initialization of the therapy. Catheter insertion is performed by the nephrologist and guided by ultrasound. The nursing staff is responsible for setting up of the circuit and the filter, and for programming the monitor according to the nephrologist prescription.

Modern CRRT platforms, such as Primaflex monitors, allow for a friendly, safe and easy-to-use configuration and programming. Also, high-precision fluid monitoring and its easy interpretation on the screen with updated information allow for optimal therapy monitoring and to achieve personalized treatment to reach dosage targets and fluid balance. RTS uses bicarbonate replacement fluids and filters with high permeability and adsorptive properties; dosage and modality are clearly defined in the RTS CRRT protocols.

The specialized RTS CRRT team has established parameters for optimal care and quality goals (**Table 7**).

CRRT initiation	**CRRT delivery dose**	**Reach ultrafiltration**
Target < 3 hours	Target > 25 ml/kg/h	Target > 80%
KPI > 90%	KPI 80%	KPI > 90%
Downtime	**Filter life time**	**Access alarms**
Target < 15%	Target > 30 h	Target < 5 in 24 h
KPI 90%	KPI > 90%	KPI > 90%

KPI: key performance indicator.

Table 7. CRRT quality indicators.

RTS has a policy of no anticoagulation in patients with high and medium risk of hemorrhage. Over the years, the nursing staff has gained experience in circuit maintenance. In highly experienced groups in RTS, the average survival time of the CRRT filter is up to 36 hours; 60% of the filters do not require anticoagulation in addition to the usual prophylaxis used for ICU patients. The heparin protocol is used for filters with less than 24 hours of lifespan; the dose is adjusted to maintain aTTP of 45 s and vTTP 65 s, the nursing team is responsible for sampling the circuit and reporting results to the specialist. The performance of the filter is evaluated daily, determined by the ratio between nitrogen loss in the ultrafiltrate and the blood urea nitrogen, to anticipate any circuit change when the result is less than 80%.

The nephrologist visits patients with CRRT two or three times a day, assesses changes in the general health of the patient, organic dysfunction, fluid balance, analysis of laboratory tests, organ supports and clinical concerns of the consultant of the UCI. The adjustment to the CRRT prescription is discussed with the ICU staff to maintain consistency in the patient treatment and to understand, in concert, planned clinical targets. Hemodynamic, ventilatory, and fluid monitoring should be guaranteed during the CRRT. The decision to wean off the renal support is evaluated at least daily, considering diuresis, markers of clearance and improvement of multi-organ failure. Close monitoring during the next 6 hours after the suspension of CRRT is a regular practice; some patients need control laboratories to maintain a safe weaning. All patients are followed up according to the nephrologist's clinical criteria.

The RET nursing staff is responsible for therapy maintenance and care for the circuit and the filter lifespan. They keep hourly records of circuit parameters such as pressures, flows, air detection in the circuits; and changes out of the expected parameters are reported to the nephrologist. The nursing staff is trained to solve regular alerts and to follow simple algorithms prior to the nephrologist intervention. A continuing education program and a periodic evaluation of protocols adherence are given to the nursing staff to guarantee homogeneous experience levels. Records are analyzed, and coagulation cases are discussed on a daily basis.

Additional clinical parameters are recorded on the CRRT flowsheet and in the CRRT EMR as well (**Figure 1**).

Monthly, the results of the program are discussed in the CNP committee, consisting of the nephrology director, the nursing leader, the medical team and the clinical operations manager. The Prismaflex CRRT management report is obtained directly from the Prismaflex monitors through the Sharesource connect platform. It collects and analyzes all the therapy parameters at each center (**Figure 2**). The results obtained are contrasted with the established CRRT quality indicators, targets and KPI. The CNP committee also analyzes survival, renal recovery, adverse events as well as the cost-effectiveness of the evaluated period. This is how quality improvement plans for the teams are defined.

4.2. Audit results

Patients older than 18 years who underwent CRRT for renal indication, during ICU stay were included in the analysis of audit results. Therapy less than 24 hours, mortality within the first 24 hours of treatment and patients with missing information were excluded from the analysis. Only data from the first intervention period were included. The population was characterized

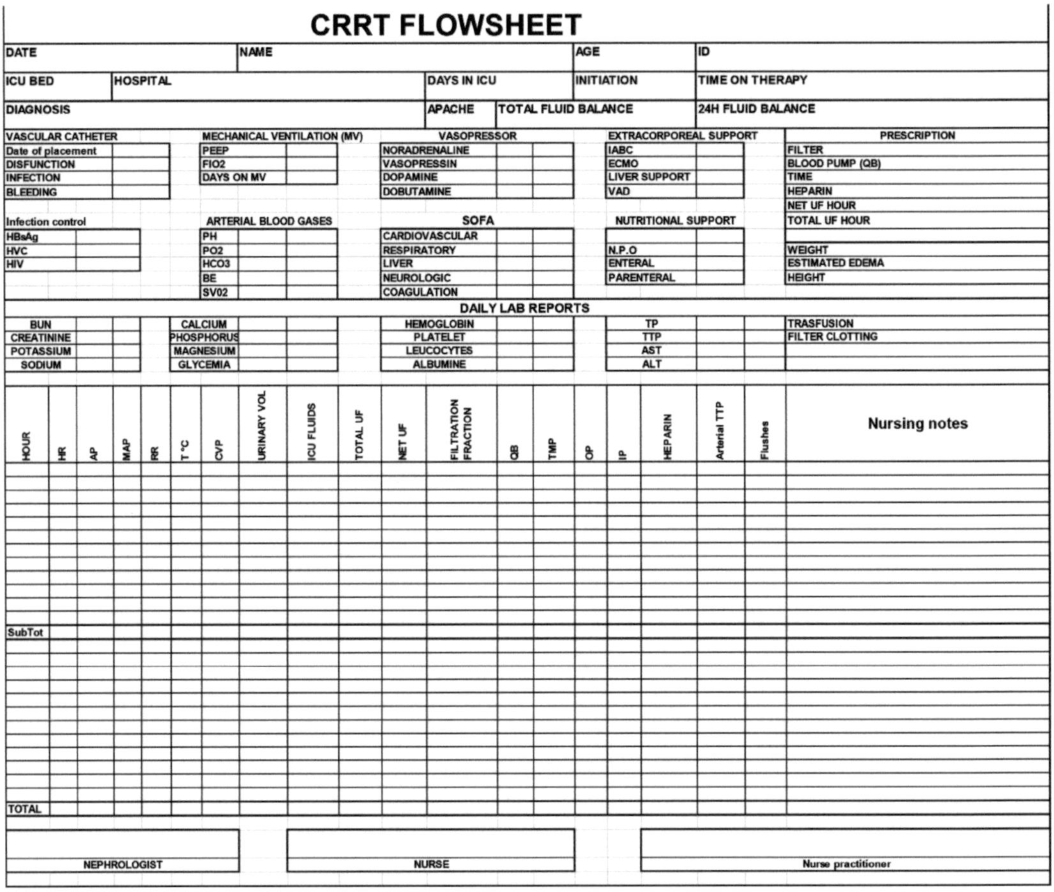

CRRT FLOWSHEET

DATE | NAME | AGE | ID
ICU BED | HOSPITAL | DAYS IN ICU | INITIATION | TIME ON THERAPY
DIAGNOSIS | APACHE | TOTAL FLUID BALANCE | 24H FLUID BALANCE

VASCULAR CATHETER: Date of placement, DISFUNCTION, INFECTION, BLEEDING
MECHANICAL VENTILATION (MV): PEEP, FIO2, DAYS ON MV
VASOPRESSOR: NORADRENALINE, VASOPRESSIN, DOPAMINE, DOBUTAMINE
EXTRACORPOREAL SUPPORT: IABC, ECMO, LIVER SUPPORT, VAD
PRESCRIPTION: FILTER, BLOOD PUMP (QB), TIME, HEPARIN, NET UF HOUR, TOTAL UF HOUR, WEIGHT, ESTIMATED EDEMA, HEIGHT

Infection control: HBsAg, HVC, HIV
ARTERIAL BLOOD GASES: PH, PO2, HCO3, BE, SV02
SOFA: CARDIOVASCULAR, RESPIRATORY, LIVER, NEUROLOGIC, COAGULATION
NUTRITIONAL SUPPORT: N.P.O, ENTERAL, PARENTERAL

DAILY LAB REPORTS
BUN, CREATININE, POTASSIUM, SODIUM
CALCIUM, PHOSPHORUS, MAGNESIUM, GLYCEMIA
HEMOGLOBIN, PLATELET, LEUCOCYTES, ALBUMINE
TP, TTP, AST, ALT
TRASFUSION, FILTER CLOTTING

HOUR | HR | AP | MAP | RR | T °C | CVP | URINARY VOL | ICU FLUIDS | TOTAL UF | NET UF | FILTRATION FRACTION | QB | TMP | OP | IP | HEPARIN | Arterial TTP | Flushes | Nursing notes

SubTot

TOTAL

NEPHROLOGIST | NURSE | Nurse practitioner

Figure 1. CRRT flowsheet. PEEP: positive end expiratory pressure. FiO_2: fraction of inspired oxygen. IABC: intra-aortic balloon counterpulsation. ECMO: extracorporeal membrane oxygenation. VAD: ventricular assist device. HR: heart rate. AP: arterial pressure. MAP: mean arterial pressure. RR: respiratory rate. T: temperature. CVP: central venous pressure. UF: ultrafiltration. Qb: blood flow. TMP: transmembrane pressure. OP: circuit outlet pressure. IP: circuit inlet pressure.

by age, sex, indication of CRRT, AKI etiology, and length of hospital stay. Some clinical characteristics were recorded at the therapy start, including serum creatinine, ureic nitrogen, pH, lactic acid, cardiovascular SOFA, vasopressor, mechanical ventilator, and fluid balance. CRRT technique such as modality, dose, and net UF within the first 24 hours were recorded. Inhospital mortality and renal function recovery, defined as dialysis independency at of hospital discharge, were analyzed.

In both of the centers participating in the audit, 265 patients underwent CRRT during the period described. **Table 8** shows the clinical characteristics of the patient. Sepsis, cardiovascular disease, and postoperative abdominal states were the main causes of acute kidney injury. The most frequent CRRT indications were metabolic acidosis, hyper-azotemia and fluid overload in 46, 34.7, and 10.9% of patients, respectively (**Figure 3**). The majority of patients

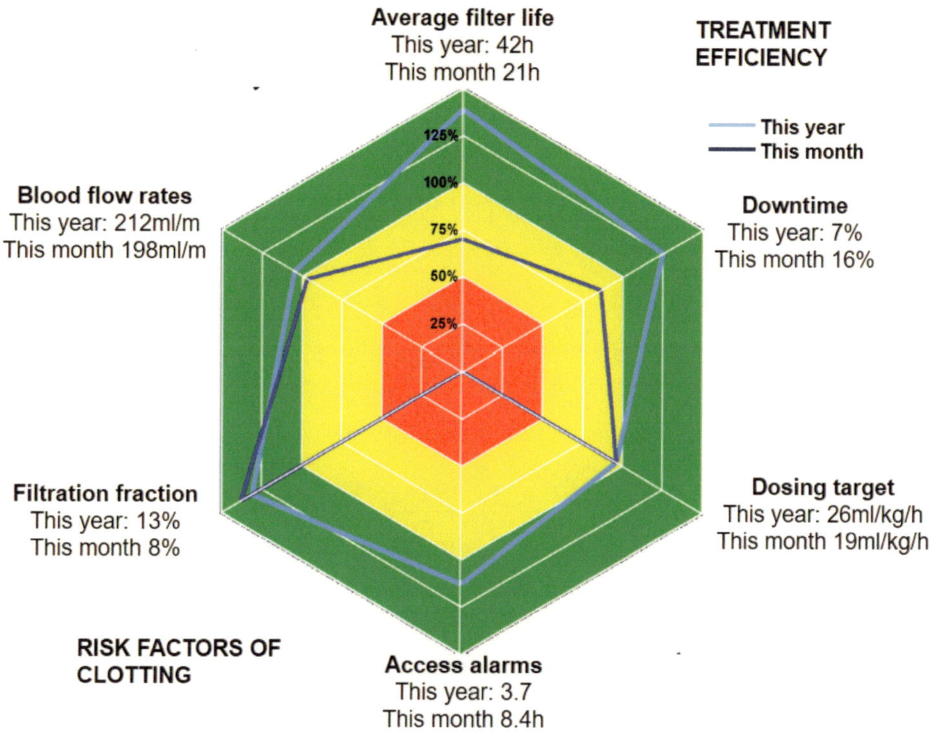

Figure 2. Prismaflex CRRT management report.

(74.7%) had 3 and 4 points of cardiovascular SOFA at CRRT beginning. The mean total SOFA was 10.3, with almost half of the patients (43.4%) with a score equal to or greater than 11.

Continuous veno-venous hemofiltration (CVVH) was the preferred CRRT modality predominantly in the predilution mode. The average of fluid balance at therapy start was 9.5 L (range −2.3 to 69 L) and the net ultrafiltration in the first 24 hours of CRRT was 1387 mL. Hospital mortality rate was similar to worldwide reports (63%), but we found a higher rate of renal recovery in the patients who survived (82%) (**Figure 4**). The average time on mechanical ventilation was 7 days with 31 days of hospital length of stay.

4.3. Economic analysis of the audit

The cost-effectiveness of continuous renal replacement therapies has been questioned in different health systems. Information on the economic impact of a service model by an external provider has not been well studied. Audit results in the renal recovery have motivated the development of an analytical model of Markov that adapts a previously validated model to our reality, in a time horizon of 5–10 years and subsequent simulation of a hypothetical cohort of 1000 patients. Health costs (COP) and adjusted life quality (QALY) were compared between intermittent hemodialysis and CRRT provided by a renal emergency team (**Table 9**) [54].

Characteristic	Number (%)
Gender—number (%)	
Male	172 (64.9)
Female	93 (35.1)
Age—years	64.7 (18–92)
Acute kidney injury etiology	
Sepsis	148 (55.8)
Cardiovascular disease	58 (21.9)
Abdominal postoperative state	31 (11.7)
Coronary artery bypass grafting	17 (6.4)
Autoimmune disease	5 (1.9)
Trauma	4 (1.5)
Nephrotoxicity	2 (0.8)
Vasopressor therapy at CRRT initiation	213 (80.4)
Cardiovascular SOFA score—number (%)	
0	53 (20)
1	5 (1.9)
2	9 (3.4)
3	77 (29.1)
4	121 (45.7)
Characteristic	**Mean (SD)**
Total SOFA score	10.3 (3.89)
pH	7.24 (0.12)
Bicarbonate (HCO_3)—mmol/L	16.4 (4.98)
Base excess (BE)	−9.09 (6.89)
Lactate (mmol/L)	3.3 (3.59)
Serum creatinine (mg/dL)	3.8 (4.14)
BUN (mg/dL)	63.9 (31.75)
Delivered dose (mL/kg/h)	26.9 (7.02)
Fluid balance at CRRT initiation (L)	9.5 (11.78)
Net ultrafiltration within the first 24 hours (L)	1.3 (1.87)

Table 8. CRRT patient characteristics (265 patients).

The results of the economic analysis showed that CRRT performed by a highly specialized external provider with optimal renal recovery results was a dominant alternative when compared with IHD (**Figure 5**). The results were maintained after a sensitivity analysis varying

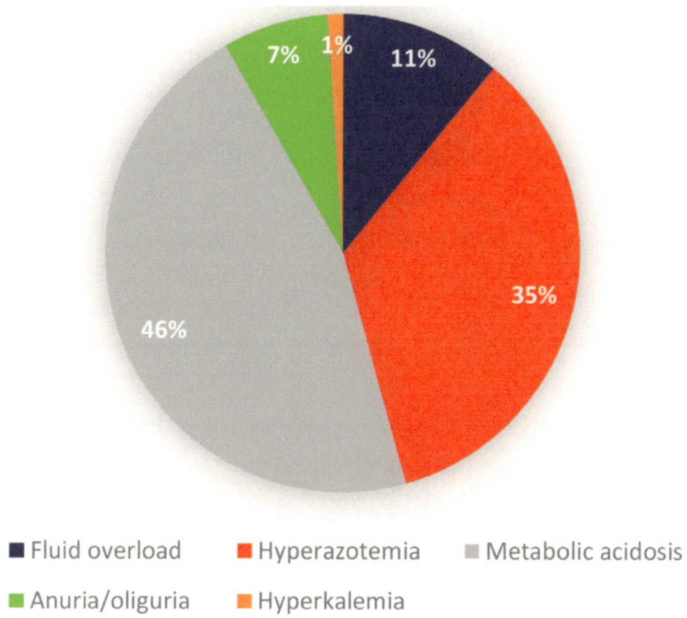

Figure 3. CRRT indications.

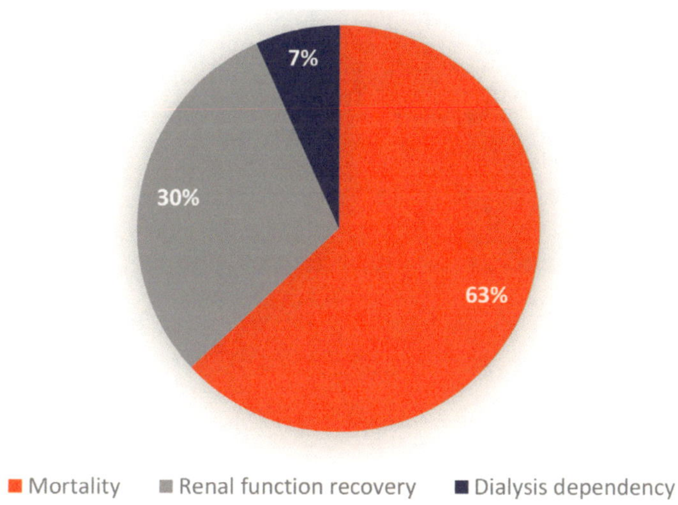

Figure 4. Inhospital outcomes.

costs, time on therapy, and mortality. The experience of a specialized CRRT service model such as RTS increases the net monetary benefit in emerging countries and invites other healthcare systems to challenge the adoption of high-quality service models.

		5% discount		
		Intermittent	Continuous therapy	Difference
Total cost (COP)		IRRT	CRRT	
	1 year	10,442,981,398	7,646,696,331	−2,796,285,067
	5 years	26,847,707,264	15,079,774,140	−11,767,933,123
	10 years	38,715,397,630	20,959,366,355	−17,756,031,275
Total QALY				
	1 year	210	231	21.3
	5 years	670	745	75.1
	10 years	992	1103	111.0

Table 9. Base case results (Cohort 1.000).

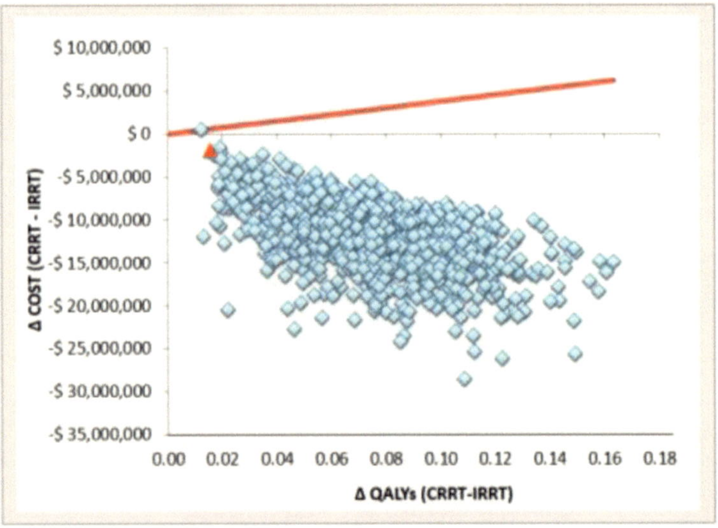

Figure 5. Probabilistic analysis.

5. Conclusion

In this chapter, we described the characteristics of our renal emergency team model and the rationale of a CRRT specialized team. Understanding how the alarm system works, being ready to act, carrying out timely interventions, developing a quality improvement program, and being able to have two-way learning between ICU and the nephrology team are part of the key aspects for success. From our experience, we showed the results of two centers of excellence where our model operates in Colombia, obtaining high clinical results, high-quality standards, and improvement in renal recovery. The population analyzed was critically ill, with high rates of multi-organ dysfunction and hemodynamic instability. The protocols used allowed a good filter life and an optimal delivered therapy dose as per international recommendations.

Sepsis is still the disease most associated with acute kidney injury as well as postoperative conditions and cardiovascular failure. Severe metabolic acidosis, positive fluid balances, and the requirement for vasoactive support continue to be frequent conditions during the initiation of CRRT. Although azotemia is the second most frequent indication in our registry, it is moderate and usually involves some of the formerly mentioned factors. Absolute indications for starting dialysis are rare in our registry. The burden of severe acute kidney injury remains important, not only because of the consumption of hospital resources but also because of the long-term prognosis and the consequent dependence on dialysis. Providing an adequate renal care system in the hospital aligned with the renal recovery policies should be part of the interest and approach of all the stakeholders in the healthcare system. Decisions in health economics and care models in extracorporeal therapies should integrate these elements.

Acknowledgements

We want to acknowledge the work done by the critical nephrology team of RTS Colombia (SER), especially the invaluable contributions provided by Andres Arboleda, MD, for the development of the CRRT model, and our nurse leaders Amanda Castro and Amelida Rincon.

Conflict of interest

Dr. Jorge Echeverri wrote this chapter while being the nephrology director of RTS Central Military Hospital. He is currently the global medical director for Acute Therapies at Baxter Healthcare Corporation.

Author details

Jorge Echeverri[1]*, Carolina Larrarte[1] and Manuel Huerfano[2]

*Address all correspondence to: jorge_echeverry@baxter.com

1 RTS Central Military Hospital, Bogotá, Colombia

2 RTS Renal Emergency Team, Bogota, Colombia

References

[1] Lameire NH, Bagga A, Cruz D, De Maeseneer J, Endre Z, Kellum JA, et al. Acute kidney injury: An increasing global concern. Lancet. 2013;**382**(9887):170-179. DOI: 10.1016/S0140-6736(13)60647-9

[2] Mehta RL, Cerdá J, Burdmann EA, Tonelli M, García-García G, Jha V, et al. International Society of Nephrology's 0by25 initiative for acute kidney injury (zero preventable deaths by 2025): A human rights case for nephrology. Lancet. 2015;**385**(9987):2616-2643. DOI: 10.1016/S0140-6736(15)60126-X

[3] Mehta RL, Burdmann EA, Cerdá J, Feehally J, Finkelstein F, García-García G, et al. Recognition and management of acute kidney injury in the International Society of Nephrology 0by25 Global Snapshot: A multinational cross-sectional study. Lancet. 2016;**387**(10032): 2017-2025. DOI: 10.1016/S0140-6736(16)30240-9

[4] Susantitaphong P, Cruz DN, Cerda J, Abulfaraj M, Alqahtani F, Koulouridis I, et al. Acute kidney injury advisory group of the American society of nephrology. World incidence of AKI: A meta-analysis. Clinical Journal of the American Society of Nephrology. 2013;**8**(9): 1482-1493. DOI: 10.2215/CJN.00710113

[5] Hoste EA, Bagshaw SM, Bellomo R, Cely CM, Colman R, Cruz DN, et al. Epidemiology of acute kidney injury in critically ill patients: The multinational AKI-EPI study. Intensive Care Medicine. 2015;**41**(8):1411-1423. DOI: 10.1007/s00134-015-3934-7

[6] Coca SG, Singanamala S, Parikh CR. Chronic kidney disease after acute kidney injury: A systematic review and meta-analysis. Kidney International. 2012;**81**:442-448. DOI: 10.1038/ki.2011.379

[7] Omotoso BA, Abdel-Rahman EM, Xin W, et al. Acute kidney injury (AKI) outcome, a predictor of long-term major adverse cardiovascular events (MACE). Clinical Nephrology. 2016;**85**:1-11. DOI: 10.5414/CN108671

[8] Collister D, Pannu N, Ye F, James M, Hemmelgarn B, Chui B, et al. Alberta kidney disease network. Health care costs associated with AKI. Clinical Journal of the American Society of Nephrology. 2017;**12**(11):1733-1743. DOI: 10.2215/CJN.00950117

[9] Douvris A, Malhi G, Hiremath S, McIntyre L, Silver SA, Bagshaw SM, et al. Interventions to prevent hemodynamic instability during renal replacement therapy in critically ill patients: A systematic review. Critical Care. 2018;**22**(1):41. DOI: 10.1186/s13054-018-1965-5.

[10] Bagshaw SM, Berthiaume LR, Delaney A, Bellomo R. Continuous versus intermittent renal replacement therapy for critically ill patients with acute kidney injury: A meta-analysis. Critical Care Medicine. 2008;**36**:610-617. DOI: 10.1097/01.CCM.0B013E3181611F552

[11] Shetz M, Lauwers P, Ferdinande P, Van de Walle J. The use of continuous arteriovenous haemofiltration in intensive care medicine. Acta Anaesthesiologica Belgica. 1984;**35**:67-78

[12] Craig MA, Depner TA, Chin E, Tweedy RL, Hokana L, Newby-Lintz M. Implementing a continuous renal replacement therapies program. Advances in Renal Replacement Therapy. 1996;**3**(4):348-350

[13] Gilbert RW, Caruso DM, Foster KN, Canulla MV, Nelson ML, Gilbert EA. Development of a continuous renal replacement program in critically ill patients. American Journal of Surgery. 2002;**184**(6):526-532

[14] Uchino S, Kellum JA, Bellomo R, Doig GS, Morimatsu H, Morgera S, et al. Acute renal failure in critically ill patients: A multinational, multicenter study. Journal of the American Medical Association. 2005;**294**(7):813-818

[15] Clark WR, Ding X, Qiu H, Ni Z, Chang P, Fu P, et al. Renal replacement therapy practices for patients with acute kidney injury in China. PLoS One. 2017;**12**(7):e0178509. DOI: 10.1371/journal.pone.0178509

[16] Bagshaw SM, Darmon M, Ostermann M, Finkelstein FO, Wald R, Tolwani AJ, et al. Current state of the art for renal replacement therapy in critically ill patients with acute kidney injury. Intensive Care Medicine. 2017;**43**(6):841-854. DOI: 10.1007/s00134-017-4762-8

[17] Ronco C, Bellomo R. Critical care nephrology: The time has come. Nephrology, Dialysis, Transplantation. 1998;**13**:264-267

[18] Endre ZH. The role of nephrologist in the intensive care unit. Blood Purification. 2017;**43** (1–3):78-81. DOI: 10.1159/000452318

[19] Askenazi DJ, Heung M, Connor MJ Jr, Basu RK, Cerdá J, Doi K, et al. Optimal role of the nephrologist in the intensive care unit. Blood Purification. 2017;**43**(1–3):68-77. DOI: 10.1159/000452317.

[20] Meersch M, Schmidt C, Hoffmeier A, Van Aken H, Wempe C, Gerss J, et al. Prevention of cardiac surgery-associated AKI by implementing the KDIGO guidelines in high risk patients identified by biomarkers: The PrevAKI randomized controlled trial. Intensive Care Medicine. 2017;**43**(11):1551-1561. DOI: 10.1007/s00134-016-4670-3

[21] Göcze I, Jauch D, Götz M, Kennedy P, Jung B, Zeman F, et al. Biomarker-guided intervention to prevent acute kidney injury after major surgery: The prospective randomized BigpAK study. Annals of Surgery. 2018;**267**(6):1013-1020. DOI: 10.1097/SLA.0000000000002485

[22] Ricci Z, Romagnoli S, Ronco C, La Manna G. From continuous renal replacement therapies to multiple organ support therapy. Contributions to Nephrology. 2018;**194**:155-169. DOI: 10.1159/000485634

[23] Romagnoli S, Ricci Z, Ronco C. Novel extracorporeal therapies for combined renal-pulmonary dysfunction. Seminars in Nephrology. 2016;**36**(1):71-77. DOI: 10.1016/j.semnephrol.2016.01.002

[24] Kellum JA, Murugan R. Effects of non-severe acute kidney injury on clinical outcomes in critically ill patients. Critical Care. 2016;**20**:159. DOI: 10.1186/s13054-016-1295-4

[25] Grams ME, Rabb H. The distant organ effects of acute kidney injury. Kidney International. 2012;**81**(10):942-948. DOI: 10.1038/ki.2011.241

[26] Donovan AL, Aldrich JM, Gross AK, Barchas DM, Thornton KC, Schell-Chaple HM, et al. Interprofessional Care and Teamwork in the ICU. Critical Care Medicine. 2018;**46**(6):980-990. DOI: 10.1097/CCM.0000000000003067

[27] Rizo-Topete LM, Rosner MH, Ronco C. Acute kidney injury risk assessment and the nephrology rapid response team. Blood Purification. 2017;**43**(1–3):82-88. DOI: 10.1159/000452402

[28] Mortimer RH, Sewell JR, Roberton DM, et al. Lessons from the clinical support systems program: Facilitating better practice through leadership and team building. The Medical Journal of Australia. 2004;**180**:197

[29] Kee YK, Kim EJ, Park KS, Han SG, Han IM, Yoon CY, et al. The effect of specialized continuous renal replacement therapy team in acute kidney injury patients treatment. Yonsei Medical Journal. 2015;**56**(3):658-665. DOI: 10.3349/ymj.2015.56.3.658

[30] Oh HJ, Lee MJ, Kim CH, Kim DY, Lee HS, Park JT, et al. The benefit of specialized team approaches in patients with acute kidney injury undergoing continuous renal replacement therapy: Propensity score matched analysis. Critical Care. 2014;**18**(4):454. DOI: 10.1186/s13054-014-0454-8

[31] Mehran R, Nikolsky E. Contrast-induced nephropathy: Definition, epidemiology, and patients at risk. Kidney International. Supplement. 2006;**100**(100):S11-S15

[32] Zarbock A, Schmidt C, Van Aken H, Wempe C, Martens S, Zahn PK, et al. Renal-RIPC investigators: Effect of remote ischemic preconditioning on kidney injury among high-risk patients undergoing cardiac surgery: A randomized clinical trial. JAMA. 2015;**313**:2133-2141. DOI: 10.1001/jama.2015.4189

[33] Thakar CV, Arrigain S, Worley S, Yared JP, Paganini EP. A clinical score to predict acute renal failure after cardiac surgery. Journal of the American Society of Nephrology. 2005; **16**(1):162-168

[34] Kagan A, Sheikh-Hamad D. Contrast-induced kidney injury: Focus on modifiable risk factors and prophylactic strategies. Clinical Cardiology. 2010;**33**(2):62-66. DOI: 10.1002/clc.20687

[35] Prowle JR, Echeverri JE, Ligabo EV, Ronco C, Bellomo R. Fluid balance and acute kidney injury. Nature Reviews. Nephrology. 2010;**6**(2):107-115. DOI: 10.1038/nrneph.2009.213

[36] Parikh CR, Moledina DG, Coca SG, Thiessen-Philbrook HR, Garg AX. Application of new acute kidney injury biomarkers in human randomized controlled trials. Kidney International. 2016;**89**:1372-1379. DOI: 10.1016/j.kint.2016.02.027

[37] Kheterpal S, Tremper KK, Heung M, et al. Development and validation of an acute kidney injury risk index for patients undergoing general surgery: Results from a national data set. Anesthesiology. 2009;**110**(3):505-515. DOI: 10.1097/ALN.0b013e3181979440

[38] Forni LG, Dawes T, Sinclair H, Cheek E, Bewick V, Dennis M, et al. Identifying the patient at risk of acute kidney injury: A predictive scoring system for the development of acute kidney injury in acute medical patients. Nephron. Clinical Practice. 2013;**123**(3–4):143-150. DOI: 10.1159/000351509

[39] Hodgson LE, Dimitrov BD, Roderick PJ, Venn R, Forni LG. Predicting AKI in emergency admissions: An external validation study of the acute kidney injury prediction score (APS). BMJ Open. 2017;**7**(3):e013511. DOI: 10.1136/bmjopen-2016-013511

[40] Basu RK, Zappitelli M, Brunner L, Wang Y, Wong HR, Chawla LS, et al. Derivation and validation of the renal angina index to improve the prediction of acute kidney injury in critically ill children. Kidney International. 2014;**85**:659-667. DOI: 10.1038/ki.2013.349

[41] Matsuura R, Srisawat N, Claure-Del Granado R, Doi K, Yoshida T, Nangaku M, et al. Use of the renal angina index in determining acute kidney injury. Kidney International Reports. 2018;**3**(3):677-683. DOI: 10.1016/j.ekir.2018.01.013

[42] Goldstein SL, Kirkendall E, Nguyen H, Schaffzin JK, Bucuvalas J, Bracke T, et al. Electronic health record identification of nephrotoxin exposure and associated acute kidney injury. Pediatrics. 2013;**132**:e756-e767. DOI: 10.1542/peds.2013-0794

[43] Colpaert K, Hoste EA, Steurbaut K, Benoit D, Van Hoecke S, De Turck F, et al. Impact of real-time electronic alerting of acute kidney injury on therapeutic intervention and progression of RIFLE class. Critical Care Medicine. 2012;**40**:1164-1170. DOI: 10.1097/CCM.0b013e3182387a6b

[44] Cho A, Lee JE, Yoon JY, Jang HR, Huh W, Kim YG, et al. Effect of an electronic alert on risk of contrast-induced acute kidney injury in hospitalized patients undergoing computed tomography. American Journal of Kidney Diseases. 2012;**60**:74-81. DOI: 10.1053/j.ajkd.2012.02.331

[45] Hoste EA, Kashani K, Gibney N, Wilson FP, Ronco C, Goldstein SL, et al. Impact of electronic-alerting of acute kidney injury: Workgroup statements from the 15(th) ADQI consensus conference. Canadian Journal of Kidney Health and Disease. 2016;**3**:10. DOI: 10.1186/s40697-016-0101-1

[46] Benfield CB, Brummond P, Lucarotti A, Villarreal M, Goodwin A, Wonnacott R, et al. Applying lean principles to continuous renal replacement therapy processes. American Journal of Health-System Pharmacy. 2015;**72**(3):218-223. DOI: 10.2146/ajhp140257

[47] Graham P, Lischer E. Nursing issues in renal replacement therapy: Organization, manpower assessment, competency evaluation and quality improvement processes. Seminars in Dialysis. 2011;**24**(2):183-187. DOI: 10.1111/j.1525-139X.2011.00835.x

[48] Soares DM, Pessanha JF, Sharma A, Brocca A, Ronco C. Delayed nephrology consultation and high mortality on acute kidney injury: A meta-analysis. Blood Purification. 2017;**43**(1–3):57-67. DOI: 10.1159/000452316

[49] Kashani K, Ronco C. Acute kidney injury electronic alert for nephrologist: Reactive versus proactive? Blood Purification. 2016;**42**(4):323-328

[50] Kolhe NV, Reilly T, Leung J, Fluck RJ, Swinscoe KE, Selby NM, et al. A simple care bundle for use in acute kidney injury: A propensity score-matched cohort study. Nephrology, Dialysis, Transplantation. 2016;**31**(11):1846-1854

[51] Chawla LS, Davison DL, Brasha-Mitchell E, Koyner JL, Arthur JM, Shaw AD, et al. Development and standardization of a furosemide stress test to predict the severity of acute kidney injury. Critical Care. 2013;**17**:R207. DOI: 10.1186/cc13015

[52] Zarbock A, Kellum JA, Schmidt C, Van Aken H, Wempe C, Pavenstädt H, et al. Effect of early vs delayed initiation of renal replacement therapy on mortality in critically Ill patients with acute kidney injury: The ELAIN randomized clinical trial. Journal of the American Medical Association. 2016;**315**(20):2190-2199. DOI: 10.1001/jama.2016.5828

[53] Rewa OG, Villeneuve PM, Lachance P, Eurich DT, Stelfox HT, Gibney RTN, et al. Quality indicators of continuous renal replacement therapy (CRRT) care in critically ill patients: A systematic review. Intensive Care Medicine. 2017;**43**(6):750-763. DOI: 10.1007/s00134-016-4579-x

[54] Ariza JG, Barrera L, Sanabria M, Echeverri J, Huerfano M, Arboleda A, et al. Economic evaluation of dialysis dependence following renal replacement therapy for critically ill acute kidney injury patients. ISPOR 2017. Value in Health. 2017;**20**:A867. PMD30